The Back

functions, malfunctions and care

Sheila Braggins
MCS SRP

With a Foreword by Lance Twomey
BAppSc BSc (Hons) Phd
Professor of Physiotherapy
Deputy Vice Chancellor
Curtin University of Technology, Perth
Western Australia

MOSBY

Published by Mosby–Year Book Europe Limited
Printed and bound in Great Britain by The Bath Press, Avon

ISBN 0 7234 1904 3

A CIP catalogue record for this book is available from the British Library.

For full details of all Mosby–Year Book Europe Limited titles please write to Mosby–Year Book Europe Limited, Lynton House, 7–12 Tavistock Square, London WC1H 9LB, England.

Library of Congress Cataloging-in Publication Data has been applied for.

Disclaimer

All postural corrections, methods of handling, and performance of exercises are complex; they are variable from person to person and sometimes are unpredictable. The guidelines included in this book should not be followed rigidly, as they are not applicable in all situations. Complete and appropriate assessment of individual circumstances must be undertaken.

The Author and the Publisher cannot accept responsibility for any consequences which may result from decisions made upon the basis of the advice given therein and from practicing any of these actions.

Acknowledgements

This book could not have been possible without the inspiration and encouragement of my friend Desley Kettle. As Superintendent Physiotherapist in Barnet General Hospital she nudged me out of the era of heat and massage into the ever broadening horizons of modern manipulative physiotherapy. She gave me endless advice and support throughout the period of the book's growth. Thank you, Desley.

The actual idea of writing a book came from my daughters Belinda and Martha and in the two years of writing and rewriting the family's support has been boundless.

My thanks go to:

Martha for setting me off on the computer and for supplying a solid belief in the end result.

Colin for the hours and hours of his time spent chasing articles and books all over London, and for putting up with a wife immersed in another world.

Belinda who tirelessly vetted my English and the clarity of my explanations, draft by draft, with patience and unswerving enthusiasm.

Thanks also to my friend and fellow physio Jane Kember who acted as another unflinching sounding-board for ideas; to my friend and fellow author Dennis Pepper who spent hours giving me publishing and professional writing advice; to Mark Cromerford for his help with exercises and muscle imbalance; to Mandy Avery and all my friends who gave their critical and encouraging appraisals.

Thanks too to Pan Tek Arts for their help with the artwork.

Finally, I want to give a special thanks to Lance Twomey, who, having read my original manuscript, written for the general public, encouraged me to rewrite it for the health care professional and, in addition, gave his valuable time to write the foreword of this book.

Foreword

A sound knowledge of the structure and function of the back is an essential requirement for health professionals who seek to work in this area. The vertebral column is a complex structure which has to subserve a number of often contradictory functions. It is important that the back allows a large range of motions in all directions, and yet it must serve as protection for an important part of the central nervous system; it must act as a shock absorber while also serving as the axis of support for the body. These multiple functions mean that the structure of the vertebral column is necessarily complex and it is this complexity which, in the past, seems to have deterred many health professionals (including physicians) from developing a thorough understanding of its morphology.

In recent years, there has been an acceleration in our interest in and knowledge of the anatomy of the back. There is now an excellent understanding of the development, maturation and ageing of the structures of the back and a much better knowledge of how it responds to trauma and to disease. Contrary to the myths associated with back pain, the vertebral column is intrinsically strong and able to withstand most of the usual stresses of everyday life. However, twentieth century lifestyle, with its emphasis on sedentary activity does place the vertebral column at risk under certain environmental conditions. Back pain is almost universal in Western cultures and recent research has shown that when back clinics are opened in 'developing' countries, people flock to them in large numbers. At some stage during our lives, most of us will have at least one severe episode of back pain which will cause us to seek treatment from a health professional.

Sheila Braggins has with *The Back: Functions, Malfunctions and Care*, made a significant contribution to the literature on the vertebral column for health professionals. The book is an excellent summary of current views about the way in which the back functions, ages and undergoes pathological change. She makes the important distinction between the ageing process and pathological changes and does not confuse the issues involved with the two quite different processes. In particular, her views on the intervertebral disc are contemporary and she has not made the mistake, present in so much current literature, of perpetuating the myths of the past.

It is refreshing to see that, after a lifetime of professional work, a clinician has taken the opportunity to prepare a knowledgeable, readable and very applied book on a most important topic. It adds significantly to the growing literature in the area and makes an important contribution to scholarship as well as to the care which health professionals of the future will need to provide.

Professor Lance Twomey

Contents

Introduction

You and your back

Introduction

The back in the 20th century

As early as 400BC Hippocrates wrote about treating *hyboma* or acute lumbar kyphosis but low back disability is a relatively new, Western epidemic (McKenzie, 1987). Hard work and excessive lifting strains have caused injury through the millennia (how many back pains resulted from the building of Stonehenge or the Pyramids?); but today subtle stress, occurring as much in leisure as at work, is the usual root of back trouble.

In the UK, back pain accounts for the greatest loss of work hours, and 80% of the population will experience back pain at some time in their lives (Waddell, 1989). Today's lifestyle, more than any other in history, creates an insidious strain on the back, stressing the soft tissues and predisposing them to injury.

The back is at its most vulnerable in flexion, the bent forward position as in stooping or the C-shaped curve of sitting – and this is the bane of present society. Motorised transport has replaced the horse and cart, but more damagingly, it has replaced our legs. We no longer walk for the frequent short errand giving the spine a welcome exercise in the extended (arched back) position, instead we sit in vehicles. Cars, buses, trains and planes provide hours of stressful accommodation for the back.

To make matters worse the seats into which we drape our bodies may add to the aesthetics of the sitting room, the appearance of a car, or the space accommodation of an aeroplane, but they too frequently do nothing to support the back correctly. Since the 1940's thousands of gadgets and clever implements, especially electrical tools, have been developed to help us reduce the effort of work, but little attention has been paid to people's physical environment in relation to their bodies. The craftsmen of William and Mary, Queen Anne, and the early Georgians made furniture to show a closeness of functional relationship with the human body which has, until now, not been surpassed (Pheasant, 1988).

Ergonomics, the study of the often complex inter-relationship between people and their occupational, domestic, and leisure activities (Hayne, 1984) is at last having an effect on the designs for living in many areas of life. Office furniture, in particular, is being revolutionised in its design to fit the body, especially in the realm of computer work. Car seats are improving in supportive shape and adjustability. Factory environment is being scrutinised, not only from the safety angle, but also in relation to back health. The one area which seems to be lagging behind is the easy chair industry. Here, except in rare and specialist designs, luxury is still the overriding criterion.

Sitting, stooping, lifting, pulling, pushing and carrying are the everyday activities of life. When performed in flexion with no regard to the position of the back, a strain is placed on all the soft tissue structures of the vertebral column. The strain leads to alteration of tissue, which in turn leads to malfunction. Malfunction of any mechanism leads to wear on the working parts and to a vulnerability which is unable to stand up (literally in this case!) to any strain, let alone to any minor accident.

Accident can be the cause of injury at any time; the severity of the injury depends on the amount of tissue damage, not necessarily on the apparent violence of the trauma, although the two are frequently linked. Most back pain results from new use or a culmination of constant overuse, misuse and abuse which stresses and strains the soft tissues (Maitland, 1986). Sometimes the result is merely the odd niggle of pain which clears and is forgotten. At other times stress can present itself as intermittent episodes of low back pain, varying in severity, followed by months or even years of respite between attacks. Sometimes the picture is of repeated frequent episodes, each growing more intense, but each appearing to recover with or without treatment. Then it is the tiny last straw, perhaps a small unguarded movement, that finally triggers the overburdened back into an episode of acute agony which might even require surgical intervention.

Pain

In its most minor form back pain can be irritating and frustrating; in its more major manifestations the gripping, crippling pain can be of such dimensions that, for the sufferer, images of permanent disability, wheelchairs, and paralysis are all quite common, and the possibility of recovery can seem remote. Complete recovery is possible in the vast majority of cases providing that the damage is not too great, that self-treatment or therapeutic treatment is started early, and that body movements are restored to previous full mobility with back care implemented meticulously forever.

A twinge of pain can be the first warning of danger. If the trauma is minor and if there is no repetition of injury, the tissues will heal, and the pain will disappear without lasting effect. However, if the injury is repeated over and over with little chance of tissue healing, the damaged tissue becomes repeatedly assaulted with no chance of speedy recovery. The damage frequently involves soft tissue in and around the vertebrae. Injury to any tissue takes a specific time to heal and understanding the timescale of this process is extremely important. If it is underestimated one can inadvertently retraumatise by starting full activities, such as sport, too soon or, alternatively, one can be emotionally demoralised by failing to recover at an unreasonably early self-imposed date.

Repair and recovery

All injury mends with scar tissue, which is less elastic and less supple than the original tissue and, unless it is purposefully stretched back to its previous length, it will impose restrictions on full range movements to the whole area. Scarred, contracted structures will therefore always be vulnerable to any sudden stretch beyond their shortened length, even a relatively small tweak. The stretch will damage the previously-affected tissue again and new scarring will reinforce the shortening.

Inevitably, the cycle will be repeated over and over with the growing probability that other structures in the area will become stressed and injured in the increasing malfunction. Damaged tissue must be gently, firmly, but steadily stretched during the later stages of the healing process until normal full-range movements are achieved. If this is not done, there is always a danger of re-injury with less and less provocation. A rigid back is vulnerable – a supple back, like a flexible tree, is able to withstand the hurricanes of life. Full recovery is a prevention of further injury.

Back care

Back pain can originate from sudden trauma, which is often avoidable, or from gradual injury, a cumulative build-up of small damage of which we are mainly unaware, and which we can usually do something about by looking after our backs.

The essential requirements of back care are:

- an awareness of the mechanical function of the healthy back
- a knowledge of the structures most at risk and a recognition of the forces that are a danger to those structures
- an understanding of the physiological changes that take place during injury and during the healing process
- an understanding of pain, with the ability to interpret and listen to its messages
- an appreciation of and ability to act upon the aggravating and relieving postures of *one's own pain*, understanding that there are few general rules that apply universally
- an understanding of the predisposing (underlying) and precipitating (immediate) causes of back pain, especially all the risk situations
- an awareness of self-imposed back care in its entirety, at work and leisure.

Goals

The goals of this book are to help you:

- to become familiar with the working mechanism of the healthy back
- to be aware of the possible cause of injury
- to understand the physiological processes which take place at the damaged site
- to recognise the warning signs signalled by the body's pain systems
- to appreciate the abuse inflicted onthe back during everyday activities
- to learn how to avoid this abuse
- to become familiar with guidelines for postural care in situations of work and relaxation.
- to understand and assist back pain sufferers.

Physical awareness is the secret of a successful understanding of our own bodies and the indispensable tool we must possess before we can identify with the plight of others in pain. Attitudes to pain are shrouded in too many misconceptions, archaic rules and advice which, far from providing help, often lead to further misinterpretation and mishandling of many signs and symptoms.

Part 1 looks at the shape and movement of the healthy back, at the anatomy of its individual structures, and at the disorders that can occur within those structures. Damage to any of these mechanisms can result in pain, which is described from psychological, physiological, and mechanical angles. The accent of Part 1 is on understanding back function, injury and pain, relating possible signs and symptoms to everyday experience.

Part 2 looks at back care, discussing the theories behind the prevention of back stress or injury in every aspect of life, ending with suggestions for keeping fit and for seeking expert advice when it is needed.

REFERENCES

Hayne, C. (1984). Ergonomics and Back Pain, *Physiotherapy* **70**, 1.

Maitland, G.D. (1986). *Vertebral Manipulation*, 5th ed., Butterworths.

McKenzie, R. (1987). Mechanical Diagnosis and Therapy for Low Back Pain. In: Physical Therapy for the Low Back (Twomey, L.T. and Taylor, J.R., eds.) Churchill Livingstone, USA.

Pheasant, S. (1988). *Body Space. Anthropometry, Ergonomics and Design.* Taylor and Francis, London and Philadelphia.

Waddell, G. (1989). A new clinical model for the treatment of back pain. *Back Pain. New Approaches for Rehabilitation and Education*, Manchester University Press.

Part 1

Back make-up and back break-up

1. *The human back*

Form and movement

The human back is an ingenious feat of engineering. It is a rod made up of individual bones linked together, no longer slung horizontally from hips to shoulders, supported at either end as with our most ancient ape ancestors, but now standing erect, a flexible tower braced and controlled only by the fleshy tissues surrounding the bone. At the top of the tower there is not only a nodding, turning, wobbling head, but also two extremely manipulative arms which heave around objects ranging from shopping bags to grand pianos, and bags of cement to other human beings, and which force the back to be, at best, a powerful anchor and, at worst, part of the actual lever of motion.

The back is the centre of the skeleton and the rear part of the trunk or torso which contains all the vital organs, apart from the brain which is housed in the skull. The back protects these organs from attack or injury from the rear, while the arms take action to ward off danger from the front. It is the central pivot of the body, supporting the head while increasing the versatility and direction of head movements, making it possible for example, to look under a table in an upside-down position. While the arms manipulate objects from the firm anchorage provided by the back at the top of the body, the legs, carrying the torso on its way, provide locomotion and agility from below.

As the central pivot of the body, the back needs to be strong. It is symbolically recognised as the strength of the body. Just as the expression 'put your best foot forward' describes the need for greater speed, 'put your back into it' means that there is heavy work to be done. The back muscles and abdominal muscles provide the source of this great strength.

However, because of the engineering skill of its design, the solidity and strength in no way inhibit the mobility of the back which allows for movements in all directions: stooping into forward flexion; arching back into extension; sideways bending into lateral or side flexion; twisting around with both feet still, into rotation (see **1.1**).

A combination of these movements is used many times a day in common activities, often while performing heavy lifting tasks. In the simple act of picking up a suitcase a number of combined movements are involved, including a mixture of flexion, side bending and rotation, all being performed at the same time.

Television is an excellent medium for studying movement, especially through slow-motion views of athletes or gymnasts. Sport of all kinds puts

1.1

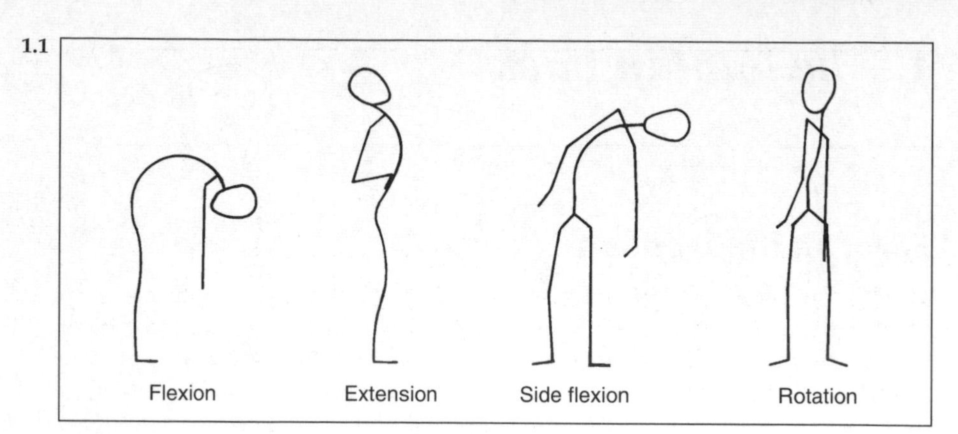

1.1 Active movements of the back

tough demands on the complicated twists and turns of which the back is capable: notice the arch, twist, backward lean and final thrust of the javelin thrower; the subtle, swaying turns of the footballer's back as he manoeuvres the ball; the full range of back movements, in all directions, used by dancers of all disciplines from disco to ballet; the thumping assault on the back as the rugby player crashes into a fellow player in a rolling tackle. It is worth noticing, too, how the weightlifter has learned to protect his back both with his belt support and, essentially, his posture. The examples are endless and the observation of any activity should help in appreciating the extent to which the back is used not only in sport but in everyday living.

Observation of other people's posture and activities is the basis for becoming aware of your own movements. The ability to analyse changes of movement, and to be aware of those changes within your own body, is an essential starting point for back care.

Before examining the detailed anatomy of the back it is important to look at the overall shape of the spine and the way in which this shape has developed.

The shaping of the curves

At birth, after lying curled up in the womb, the baby's back is in one slightly curved line. As the baby learns to hold its head up the neck curve changes, and by the time the baby is sitting up the **cervical lordosis** is an established spinal curve (**1.2**). Later, when the toddler stands, the spine adapts still further, forming a similar curve below the waist, the lumbar curve or **lumbar lordosis** (**1.3**). The end result is a prolonged S-shape, concave at the top and bottom and convex in the middle. A concave curve is a **lordosis** and a convex curve a **kyphosis**.

1.2

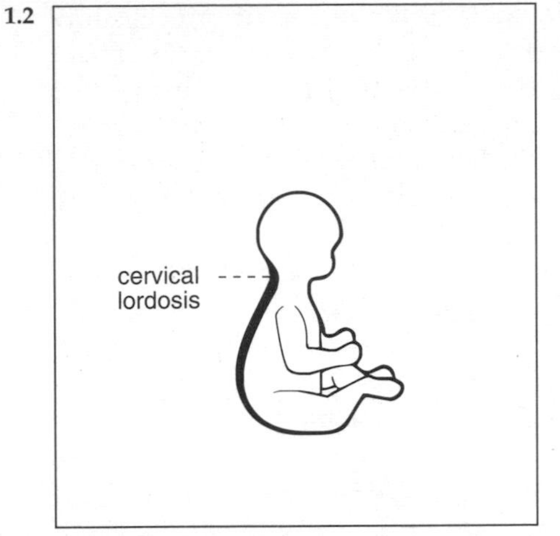

1.2 The first spinal curve

1.3

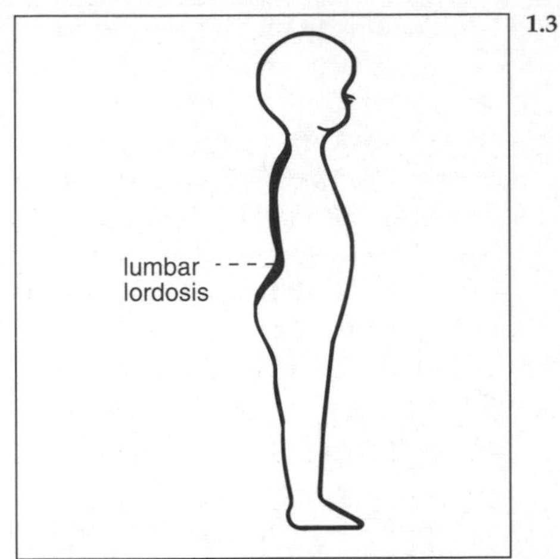

1.3 The S-shaped curve

The S-shape with its alternating curves is a valuable characteristic of the overall mechanism, giving the spine a spring-like action, with a bounce and recoil that a straight tower of bone could never provide, adding strength with adaptability. The lumbar curve is the strongest section, taking the greatest postural strain and burden of activity, but all three curves and their relationship to each other play an integral part in the function of the healthy back.

In daily living, whether standing or sitting, constantly-maintained poor posture influences the curves, either increasing them or flattening them. Any alteration of one curve creates a knock-on effect in the others. Changes in stress on the curves correspondingly place altered strain on structures unaccustomed and unprepared for the new demands. If the change of contour becomes long-lasting, permanent adaptation of the whole spine takes place, forcing tissues into new attitudes and new roles. The 'springy' facility no longer remains intact and the overall mechanism ceases to be as efficient. This is why posture is so important in back care.

An inevitable result of the permanent change of contour is a decrease in mobility. Lack of the right exercise and insufficient activity can also cause the spine to stiffen, reducing its range of movement. Rigidity results in vulnerability. The three curves need to be preserved with care, neither exaggerated nor diminished, and their flexibility maintained with exercise. The back then retains its essential characteristic of strength with mobility.

Consider again the position of the back as the centre of the skeleton. Clearly, it must not be looked at in isolation; not only do the curves affect each other, but the behaviour of the arms and legs also has a direct effect on the back. Standing with the knees bent, or conversely with them pressed back, or with the weight on one leg, alters the back position and shape of the curves. Similarly, most arm movements are stabilised by back muscle action which in turn, depending upon the dimensions of the arm activity, will generate movement of the spine. The body is a whole and, especially with regard to the skeletal structures, each part must be considered in relation to the rest. So although the curves are a component of the back, they must be viewed as a part of the entire body shape from the feet upwards. This will become clearer in the chapters on posture.

Alteration of spinal shape, injury or disease all affect the mechanisms involved with movement, the biomechanics of the spine. Disturbance of these structures can lead to pain. So the first step towards understanding back pain is understanding the **anatomy** and **physiology** of the back. The following chapters examine the role played by the bones, joints, ligaments, muscles and blood supply of the whole area.

2. The bones of the back

Bony anatomy

The spine or vertebral column runs all the way down the back from the base of the skull to the coccyx (**2.1**).

The vertebral column

The vertebral column consists of 33 vertebrae, 24 of which are individual, jointed bones placed one above the other starting from the sacrum as the base. Between each vertebra is the intervertebral disc. The vertebrae are arranged as follows:

- 7 **cervical** vertebrae of the neck
- 12 **thoracic** vertebrae in the upper trunk, sometimes called the 'dorsal' spine
- 5 **lumbar** vertebrae
- 5 **sacral** vertebrae, fused together to form the sacrum
- 4 small **coccygeal** vertebrae forming the coccyx (**2.1**).

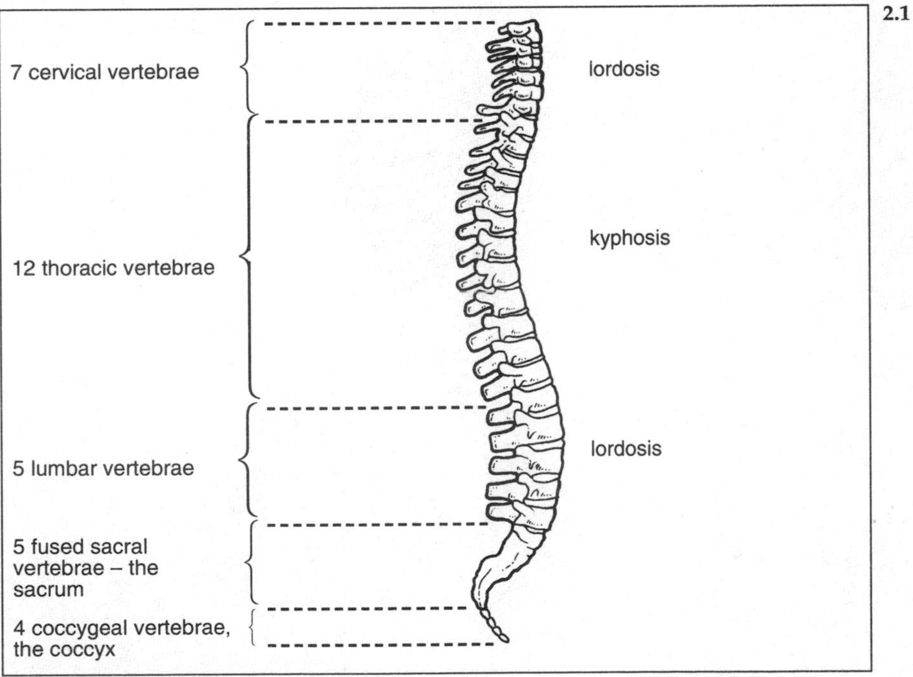

2.1 The vertebral column

Each vertebra is an irregular shape, quite complicated at first glance (**2.5**), but every knob or protrusion has a function. The vertebrae in each group are similar in design though they vary according to their position in the group and the role they play in the column as a whole. They are numbered for identification from the top down, with each vertebra given the first letter of its group name followed by the position in the group, for example, C3 would be the third cervical vertebra or L5 the fifth lumbar.

The **cervical vertebrae** are the smallest and the most mobile having only the head to support. The first two vertebrae, the **atlas** and the **axis**, are especially designed to give the greatest degree of mobility for head movements but the general morphology of all the vertebrae permits wide-ranging mobility in all directions.

The **thoracic vertebrae** are larger than the cervical. They are attached to the ribs and are adapted for this purpose. The ribs sweep round from their posterior **costo-vertebral junction** to join the **sternum** in the front,

2.2

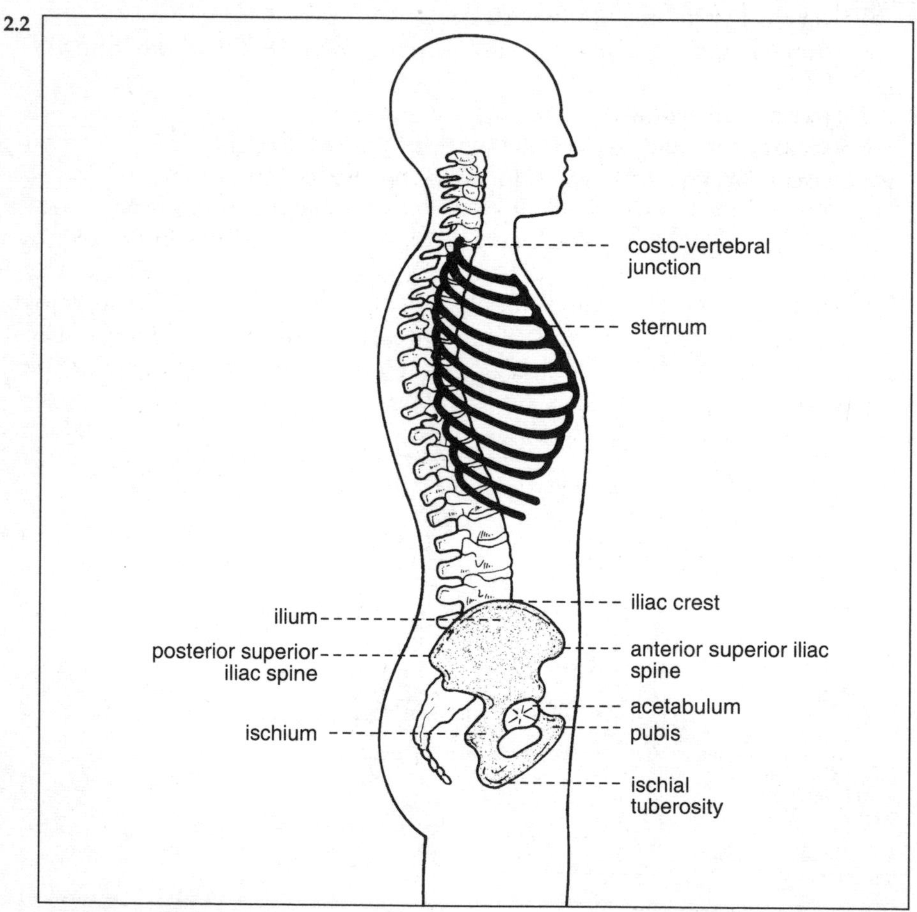

2.2 The vertebral column, ribs and hip bone

forming the rib cage which houses the heart and lungs (**2.2**). Thoracic extension and side flexion are restricted by the rib attachments.

The **lumbar vertebrae** are the biggest and toughest, designed to bear the full weight of the trunk, arms and head and to withstand the torsional strains placed upon them from the stresses of twisting trunk movements. Their greatest characteristics are their strength and mobility.

The **sacral vertebrae** are fused together to form the triangular sacrum. The upper surface of S1, the first sacral vertebra, bears the full weight of the whole upper body. This would tend to rotate the whole sacrum forwards were it not for strong controlling ligaments (Taylor and Twomey, 1987). The sacrum joins the ilium of the two hip bones on either side forming the sacro-iliac joint (**2.3**).

The **coccyx** is composed of four rudimentary vertebrae which lie below the sacrum. Their only articulation is with the apex of the sacrum. The bones are directed downwards and forwards (**2.1**).

The pelvis

The **pelvis**, which forms a basin around the lower abdomen, consists of the **sacrum**, the **coccyx** and the two **hip bones**. The hip bones are an irregular, rather contorted shape consisting of three areas: the **ilium**, the **ischium** and the **pubis,** all uniting around the **acetabulum**, the recess for articulation with the head of the **femur** (**2.2 & 2.3**). The hip bones are often confused with the **hip joint**, the latter being where the head of the femur articulates with the acetabulum (**2.3**). The actual joint is in mid-groin position where it is possible to palpate the head of the femur. The **greater trochanter** of the femur is palpable as a large bony knob at the top of the thigh, laterally.

2.3

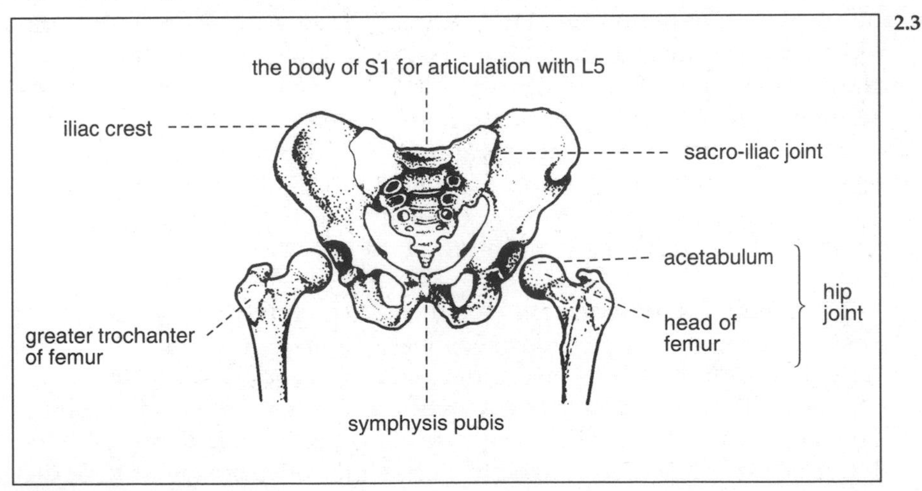

2.3 The pelvis

The **ilium** is the large portion above the acetabulum. It has an extended crest which runs from the **anterior superior iliac spine** (ASIS) in the front to the **posterior superior iliac spine** (PSIS) at the back (**2.2**). This is part of the hip bone and not the hip joint. The landmarks are easily palpable by placing the fingers and thumb around the waist, pressing down on the crest or ridge of bone below. The anterior superior iliac spine is the bony prominence palpable on each side in the front, and at the back the two dimples by the sacrum clearly denote the two posterior superior iliac spines (**2.2** and **2.3**).

The **ischium** is the lower part of the hip bone surrounding the posterior part of the acetabulum. The most obvious landmark is the **ischial tuberosity** which is palpable in the sitting position. This is the protruding bone under the buttock which can be quite painful if resting on a hard chair (**2.2**).

The **pubis** is the most anterior portion, the two pubic promontories coming together to form the **symphysis pubis** which can be palpated below the abdomen (**2.3**).

The vertebral column and pelvis meet the body's two contradictory needs – **rigidity** and **mobility** (Kapandji, 1974).

- Rigidity, supplied by the tough bones, gives strength and support to the whole back as well as protection for the important soft tissues lying in and around them.
- Mobility, resulting from the presence of many small bones and their bony articulations rather than one long pole, allows for movements in all directions.

A typical lumbar vertebra

It is beyond the scope of this book to describe each vertebral type but although they vary considerably in size and architecture, the overall principles are the same. Figure **2.4** shows L3 placed in context with the rest of the spine. A typical lumbar vertebra can be divided into **anterior** and **posterior elements** united by a bridge of bone called the **pedicle**. The anterior element is made up of the **vertebral body** and the posterior element consists of the **neural arch, laminae, spinous process, transverse processes** and **articular processes** (**2.5** and **2.6**). The two sections have very different functions, hence the complete contrast of design.

The **vertebral body** resembles a kidney-shaped drum. It is designed to sustain immense vertical loads, the whole weight of the trunk being transmitted through these solid structures. Although solid, vertebral bodies are not heavy. They are constructed of vertical and transverse beams of cancellous bone which form a rigid, lightweight cylinder, able to sustain huge longitudinal pressures as weight is transmitted from one to another (Bogduk and Twomey, 1991). The central area of the upper surface of the

2.4

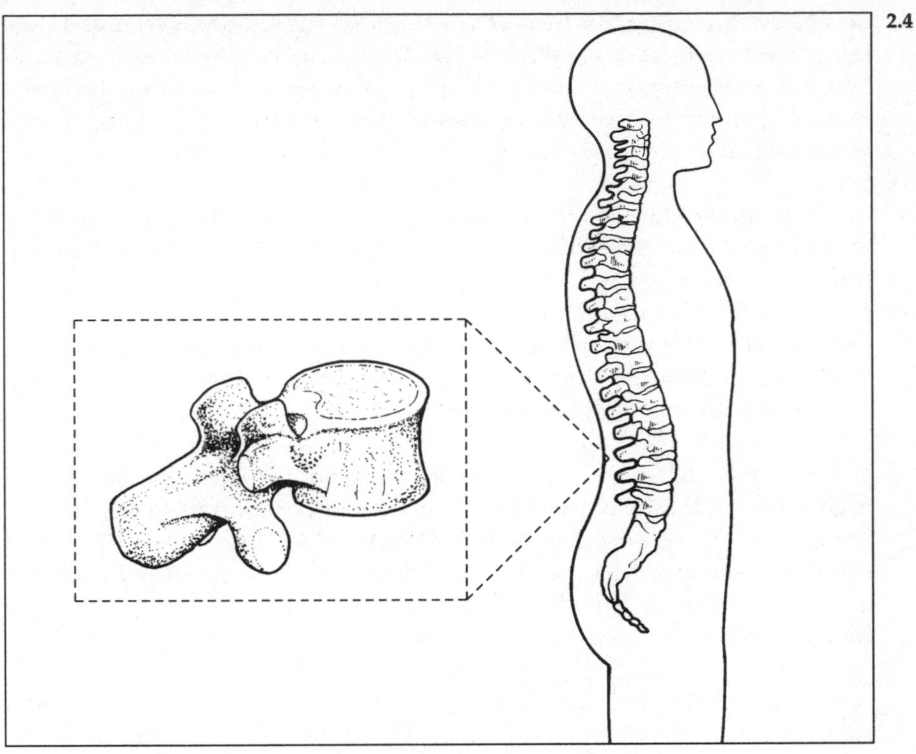

2.4 The position of L3 in the vertebral column

2.5

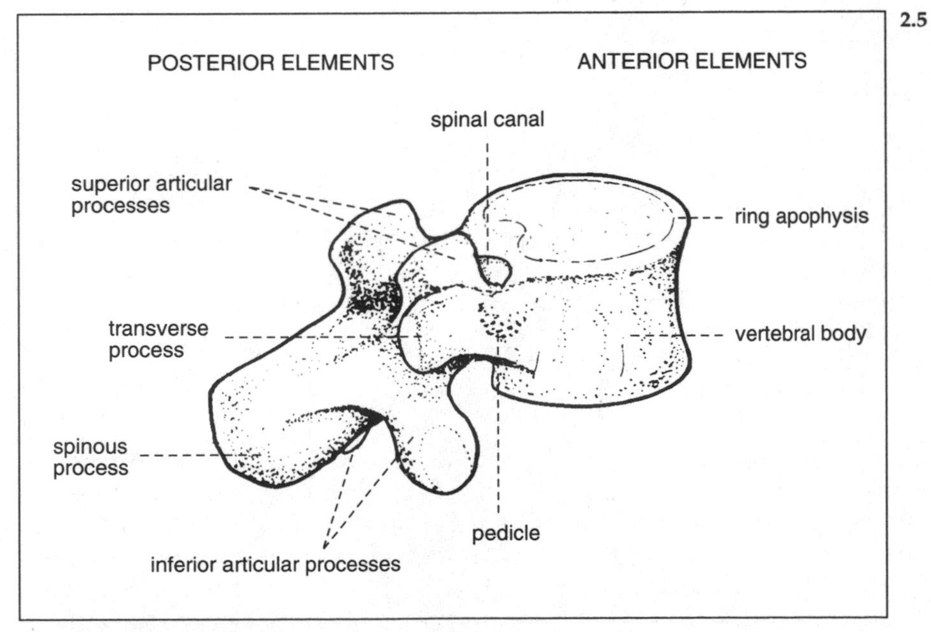

2.5 A lumbar vertebra

vertebral body is flat, perforated with minute holes and surrounded by a small rim of smoother bone on the perimeter, the ring apophysis (**2.5** and **2.6**). The perforations at the top, as well as others visible on the posterior body wall, are openings for the transmission of tiny blood vessels to the vertebral body.

The **pedicles** (**2.5**) are the connecting link between the vertebral body and the posterior elements. They are subjected to considerable bending force when the muscles of the back, attached mainly to the posterior elements, exert a downward pressure on the rear of the spine (Bogduk and Twomey, 1991). It is worth examining a vertebra to visualise these forces and relate the image to the picture of stress when the back is functioning, especially in moments of heavy lifting.

The **neural arch** is the semicircle of bone from pedicle to pedicle which together with the posterior border of the vertebral body forms the circumference of the vertebral or **spinal canal** (**2.6**). The role of the spinal canal is to give solid protection to the sensitive structures inside the canal, the spinal cord and its meninges (covering), the nerve roots and blood vessels which occupy this bony tube.

The **laminae** are two leaves of bone on the posterior border of the neural arch that eventually join together to form the **spinous process**. As the spinous process is an area of considerable muscular attachment, any force exerted upon it must be transmitted through the lamina.

2.6

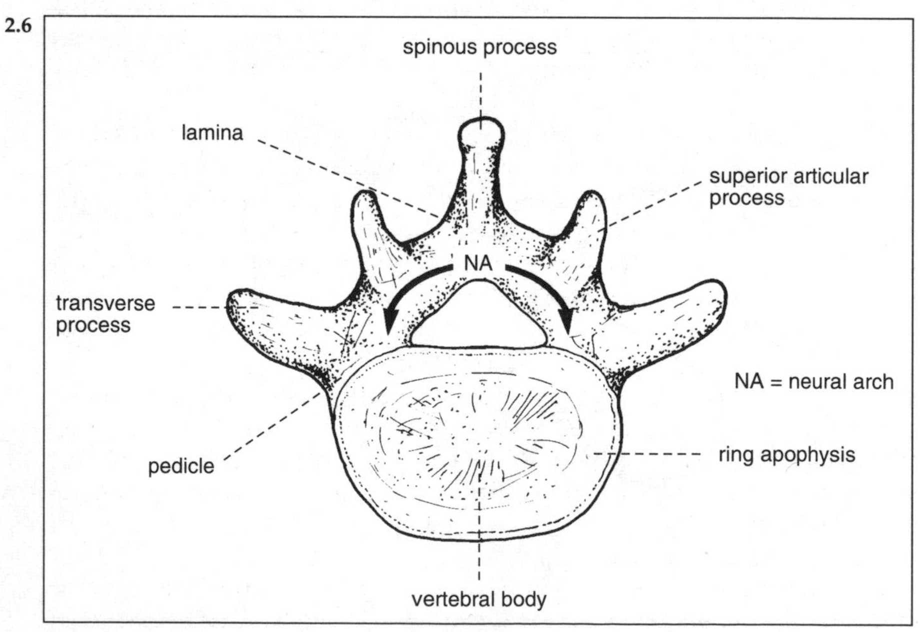

2.6 A lumbar vertebra viewed from above

The **spinous process** is the rounded projection that is palpable from one vertebra to another all down the back (**2.5**).

The **transverse processes** project laterally on either side from the junction of the pedicle and lamina. Together with the spinous process they provide areas for muscle and ligament attachments. They are the levers of the spine on which the muscle pulleys operate.

The **articular processes** – superior and inferior – are the vital joint-forming elements of the vertebrae. The inferior articular processes of one vertebra lock onto the superior articular processes of the vertebra below to form the **zygapophyseal joints** (the Z joints), sometimes called the facet joints (see Chapter 3, p. 31).

The **intervertebral foramen** (IVF) is an opening which only becomes apparent when two vertebrae are articulated (see **3.3 p. 33**). On an individual vertebra the upper and lower half of the foramen appear merely as two unnamed notches between the articular processes and the vertebral body. As soon as the motion segment is articulated they form the pear-shaped circumference of the IVF. The IVF is the vital and important passageway for the **spinal nerve**, the **sinuvertebral** nerve and **blood vessels** entering and leaving the canal. Considerable trouble can occur at this opening.

The structure of bone

Bone is a uniquely versatile tissue combining strength, elasticity and adaptability (Darby, 1992). It moulds its structure to accommodate long-term stress and is continually remodelling and renewing itself by the processes of osteoclastic resorption and osteoblastic formation (ibid).

Most bones consist of two definite types, **compact bone** and **cancellous bone**. In long bones the shaft is composed of compact bone with the ends of the bone made up of more soft, spongy cancellous bone. In the vertebrae the vertebral bodies are made up of cancellous bone, covered by a layer of compact bone. Bones are enclosed by a tough outer covering, **the periosteum**. This contains nutrient arteries which nourish the bone cells (Johnston, 1945).

Compact bone contains thousands of **Haversian systems** held together by interstitial and circumferential lamellae; cancellous bone is made up of web-like formations of spaces filled with red marrow, the spaces being separated by **trabeculae**, bony projections which give bones their strength (Mourad, 1991).

The Haversian System is composed of four parts: **lamellae, lacunae** (small cavities filled with osteocytes), **canaliculi** and the **Haversian canal** (a channel containing blood vessels) (ibid).

Bony disorders

Trauma, disease and deformity are the three main bony disorders.

Trauma

Trauma to bone is usually related to accident in sport or transport, in falls or in assault of one kind or another. Direct trauma to bone can cause damage at the point of impact or take the form of force thrust through the bony structure. Like most healthy bone the vertebrae are tough but they can, like all bone, be fractured. A fracture is a partial or complete break in a bone; it can range from a mere crack to complete shattering of the bone. Mourad (1991) gives very clear descriptions of types of fractures and the complications which may ensue.

Vertebral fractures:

- **Avulsion fractures;** sudden twisting movements with thrust or great pressure behind them, as in road accidents or whiplash injuries, can avulse small particles of bone at the junction of ligament or muscle attachments on any of the processes.
- **Compression fractures** of the vertebral body can be sustained by a fall from a height, perhaps landing on the base of the spine, or from a weight falling on the shoulders, or as a result of vertical force such as ejection from a pilot's seat (Porter, 1986). Such fractures can occur in youth and may not be discovered until later in life when for one reason or another X-rays of the spine are taken. They sometimes result in the vertebral body becoming wedge-shaped which may in turn lead to deformity (see 'scoliosis', p. 23 and 'kyphosis', p. 25).

The danger of spinal fracture lies in the possible damage to neural tissue both in the vertebral canal and in the intervertebral foramen (see Chapter 6, p. 80); if the spinal canal is already narrow (see spinal stenosis, p. 25), a flexion deformity which follows a compression fracture may cause critical compression of the spinal cord with resulting paraplegia (Porter, 1986). Neurological damage is lessened if the posterior elements avoid injury. Generally a compression fracture without bony injury to pedicles, Z joints or lamina is not considered to be a serious injury (ibid). A simple fracture with no displacement should heal well with little resulting discomfort. Fractures are maintained in good position by means of plaster of Paris splinting, traction, external fixation, internal fixation, functional bracing or a combination of these (Mourad, 1991; Thomas, 1992).

The process of injury and healing in fractures

The process of injury and healing in a fracture can be divided into three periods:

- **Inflammatory phase:** The inflammatory phase starts immediately with bleeding into the site causing a haematoma to develop around the bone ends. A clot is formed and osteocytes at the bone ends die as they are deprived of nutrients (Mourad, 1991). The presence of necrotic cells sets up an inflammatory response accompanied by vasodilation and oedema. Cells migrate into the area – fibroblasts, lymphocytes, macrophages and osteoblasts from the bone itself – and begin to form new bone. (ibid). The haematoma becomes organised by the fibroblasts forming granulation tissue, capillary buds develop and invade the area, collagen is laid down and calcium is deposited in the collagen network (Mourad, 1991; Thomas, 1992).

- **Repair phase:** Osteocytes form bony trabeculae according to the lines of force or stress in the bone and within one to two weeks after injury callus begins to appear. Callus is made up of immature woven bone and does not have the sophisticated structure of mature bone, which is made up of lamellae, interlaced by the microscopic tubules of the Haversian system (Thomas, 1992). As the purpose of callus is to prevent relative movements of bone ends, it continues to form only until it is strong enough to prevent movement (ibid). Production of callus is therefore initiated and maintained by movement. If there is no movement at all, then no callus will form; if there is too much movement it will continue to grow in an attempt to stop it. Callus is a 'one-off' response. If it does not occur within a few weeks of injury it will not occur at all (ibid).
- **Remodelling phase:** Once the movement at the fracture ends has been brought to rest by callus, the slower process of remodelling begins. Osteoclasts aid in resorbing poorly-formed or superfluous trabeculae, and the woven bone of the callus-forming phase is replaced by mature bone. The remodelling process is directed by the pattern of stress to optimise the strength of the bone (Thomas, 1992). There is no definite moment of fracture union. The clinician uses the X-ray appearance, professional experience, the extent of the original injury and the presence or absence of pain to decide when weight bearing can take place.

In normal physiological bone healing, the callus response occurs in the first two or three weeks and can continue for a few months, and remodelling begins during the first five or six weeks and can continue for years (Thomas, 1992).

All fractures are extremely painful, and movement can be excruciating. In certain fractures, for example those of the pelvis, blood loss can be significant. In cases of multiple fractures metabolic changes can take place which can cause the patient to enter a catabolic state for several days (Thomas, 1992). Psychologically, fractures can be an alarming experience. Apart from the shock of injury, fear over the prognosis and bewilderment of the new experience of plasters and crutches can be quite overpowering. Patients need great support and reassurance (Thomas, 1992).

Disease

Everyone has a nagging fear that something 'nasty' is happening within the body if pain persists for any length of time, even if it is obvious that the pain started after tripping over the dog! It is important to eliminate fear, so if in doubt, discuss this with a doctor who may well ask for an X-ray. X-rays are often taken as routine before commencing any physical treatment. They do not show soft tissue injury and in most cases give no clue to the cause of pain, but they do serve to discount the presence of disease or deformity.

Describing the possible bony diseases, for example tumour, tuberculosis, Paget's disease, osteomyelitis, osteomalacia, serves no purpose in this book, particularly as physical exercises can be entirely contraindicated in certain cases. Porter (1986), Mourad (1991) and Cash (1992) all give excellent information on these diseases. However, it is important to mention two conditions that are extremely relevant to back care: osteoporosis and ageing in bone.

Osteoporosis

Osteoporosis occurs when the processes of bone resorption and new formation break down (Darby, 1992), and the balance is disturbed with resorption becoming more extensive than bone deposition (Mourad, 1991). It can be localised or general. The change in bone density, which is often associated with hormonal changes of the menopause but which also occurs in men, is responsible for considerable vertebral pain, shortened stature and sometimes bone fractures (Twomey and Taylor, 1987). It manifests in the 'dowager's hump' of elderly ladies and in the frequent femoral neck fractures of old age. Recent investigation has demonstrated that exercise not only maintains the mobility of the spine but also improves the health of the bone, actually warding off the advent of osteoporosis (Taylor and Twomey, 1987; Twomey, 1989).

Age changes in bone

Bone is a dynamic tissue, regulated by endocrine factors, nutrition and physical activity. In the ageing process changes take place which cause an overall decrease in the density of bone and a decrease in bony strength. There is loss of support in the horizontal beams of bone in the vertebral body which leads to buckling of the vertical beams (Taylor and Twomey, 1987). This creates a gradual increase of concavity of the upper and lower surfaces of the vertebral body which will be discussed later in the age changes of the motion segment (see Chapter 4, p. 48). In the past, hormonal changes and calcium deficiencies have been accentuated as the main causes, with less emphasis on the effect of physical activity (Twomey, 1989). Athletes of all ages have greater bone density than sedentary people of the same age group and it has been proved that in young adults bony atrophy (wasting) occurs in the absence of exercise, while bone hypertrophy (increased growth) follows increased levels of activity. The quantity of bone density in athletes correlates with levels of stress exerted upon their bones, for example weightlifters have greater bone density than swimmers, and elderly swimmers have greater density than inactive people of the same age group. One of the reasons why astronauts must exercise regularly in space is that a few days of gravitational weightlessness can cause them to lose massive amounts of bone density (Twomey, 1989). Facts like these underline the necessity for active exercise to be continued regularly, well into old age.

Bone disease, though rare in everyday clinical experience, can cause considerable spinal pain and can also lead to deformity.

Deformity

Deformity is more common than disease but is often a red herring in relation to pain. Many people with deformities live completely pain-free lives, unaware of anything amiss. However, deformity does provide a vulnerability which may cause structures to succumb to stress more easily than a perfect mechanism, thus becoming an indirect cause of pain.

Deformity can occur during foetal development (Taylor and Twomey, 1987), during the later growth period or as a result of accident at any age. It can also be the result of disease. It can take the form of an alteration of vertebral body shape, an inequality in the size or shape of the zygapophyseal joints, a variation in the size of the vertebral canal or any bony irregularity of any part of the vertebra, even to the fusion of two vertebrae. The following are some of the more common vertebral anomalies.

Unilateral hemivertebra

Unilateral hemivertebra is a fault in fetal development when one side of the vertebral body fails to develop; a congenital scoliosis results and developmental failure of the anterior area of the body leads to a congenital kyphosis.

Scoliosis

Scoliosis is a fault in fetal development when one side of the vertebr is an alteration in the vertical line of the spine. When viewed from behind, the spine weaves from side to side instead of growing vertically straight. There are several types of scoliosis:

- **Osteopathic** scoliosis can be created by a vertebral asymmetry which can be congenital or acquired. The wedge-shaped bone in **2.7** can result from a failure of bony development, an injury sustained in childhood (such as a fall from a horse or crashing on to the edge of a trampoline), a vertebral body fracture or from bone disease.

2.7

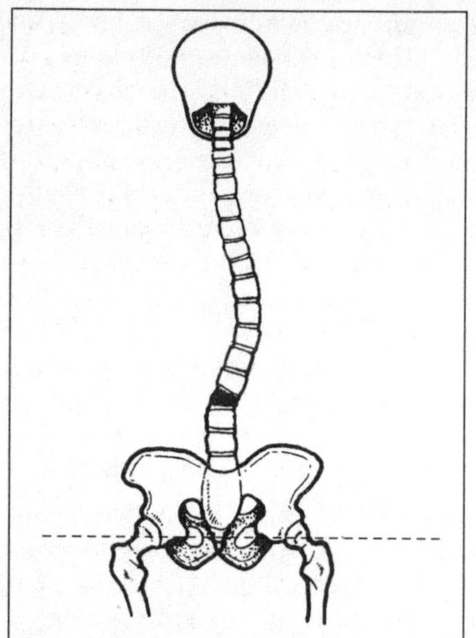

2.8

2.7 Scoliosis caused by a wedge-shaped vertebra

2.8 Scoliosis caused by a difference in leg length

- **Neuromuscular.** The spine may be normal at birth but any paralysing or neuromuscular condition, for example, cerebral palsy or one of the muscular dystrophies, can affect the stabilising spinal musculature with resulting alteration in spinal shape (Eisenstein and Draycott, 1992).
- **Idiopathic** or 'cause unknown' scoliosis is the most common type. The spine is usually normal at birth but deforms with rapid growth for reasons not understood; it develops most often in adolescent girls from the age of 10 to the end of skeletal growth (Kisner and Colby, 1990). There is usually an element of structural abnormality with some degree of rotation of the vertebrae of the thoracic spine causing a rib 'hump' (Eisenstein and Draycott, 1992). The curve is associated with a decrease or increase of thoracic kyphosis.
- **Non-structural.** Spasm in the back muscles in acute back pain can elicit a temporary scoliosis, as can habitual asymmetric postures. One of the more common causes is an alteration of the base level from which the spine grows – irregularity of pelvic symmetry or a difference in leg length. The difference in leg length (**2.8**) causes the pelvis to tip to one side, sending the spine off at a tangent like a tree growing on a bank. There need only be a difference of half a centimetre to induce a scoliosis. Leg length difference can be checked roughly in standing by either looking at the two dimples of the posterior superior iliac spines at the back of the pelvis – they should be horizontal and level with each other – or by placing both hands along the iliac crests, which should also be level with each other. Leg length can be more accurately measured in lying.

Difference in leg length is extremely common, but the cause is often unknown. Prior to the advent of poliomyelitis vaccine, shortening due to the muscle paralysis of poliomyelitis used to be a common cause (Evans and Draycott, 1992). Congenital abnormality, infection of bone and joint, fractures of long bones or overgrowth of one limb can all cause inequality of leg length. However, thousands of people are living happily, quite oblivious of the fact that they have one leg longer than the other and a slight scoliosis. After all it is really quite amazing that our cell growth instructions ever get through sufficiently accurately for any of us to end up with arms and legs of equal length – for a centipede to get them all right is even more astonishing! Correction of leg length can be made by a heel raise, although the best time for implementing this should be discussed with a doctor or therapist.

There is no statistical increase in the incidence of low back pain in scoliotic backs but disc degeneration at the apex of the curve does occur (Wiltse, 1971). The angle of the curve can be measured: less than 20° is considered to be mild but adolescents with curves greater than this are sometimes fitted for corrective braces (Kisner and Colby, 1990). In some centres this has been abandoned, not only because it is unacceptable for sensitive teenagers, but because recent studies have raised doubts about its efficacy (Eisenstein and Draycott, 1992). The non-bracing philosophy leaves the scoliosis to halt its progression spontaneously or prove its need for surgical intervention if it progresses beyond 35–40° (ibid). The condition can be an upsetting one for adolescents, especially if there is a thoracic deformity; they require considerable encouragement and support (Mourad, 1991).

Kyphotic deformity

A gross increase in thoracic kyphosis can occur in Scheuermann's disease (see Chapter 4, p. 53), from an infection or spinal injury causing a wedge-shaped vertebra, from biochemical changes (osteoporosis), from congenital abnormalities, or from degenerative changes of the discs.

Spina Bifida

Spina Bifida is a development anomaly in which the laminae of the vertebra, often L5, fail to unite. It varies in complexity from a simple deformity which causes little problem (Wiltse, 1971) to a major disruption, including splitting of the skin, neural arch and underlying neural tube with associated neurological deficits (Taylor and Twomey, 1987).

Spinal stenosis

Spinal stenosis is a narrowing of the spinal canal, the nerve root canals (see Chapter 6) or the IVF. It may be localised to one vertebra or more generalised. The narrowing may be caused by bony deformity or soft tissue deformation which could be congenital, developmental or degenerative, or a combination of all three (Arnoldi *et al.*, 1976; Crock and

Yoshizawa, 1976; Kirkaldy-Willis and McIvor, 1976). The effects range from minor irritation to major neurological or vascular changes often requiring surgical intervention.

Spondylolysis

Spondylolysis is a defect or weakening of a narrow isthmus of bone called the **pars interarticularis** which runs between the superior and inferior articular facets (Wiltse, 1971; Taylor and Twomey, 1987). If the bone breaks the lumbar column is supported at that level only by ligamentous structures. The condition in itself does not give pain but can cause instability and stress on or damage to the surrounding tissues, and can lead to spondylolisthesis.

Spondylolisthesis

Spondylolisthesis occurs when, because of a structural defect, one vertebra slips forward on the vertebra below. Forward slip of one vertebra on another, is normally resisted by the bony block of the Z joints (see above and Chapter 3, p. 31), the intact neural arch, the pedicle and by the intervertebral discs bonding together with the vertebral bodies. Articular defects and defects of the neural arch break down this mechanism and forward slip occurs most commonly at L5 or S1 (McNab, 1977). Although it presents a dramatic picture on X-ray it can be asymptomatic for a lifetime. When symptoms are present they can be those of instability (the loss of spinal ability to maintain the relationship between vertebrae without damage), root pain or pain from any compromised soft tissue. There are six clinical varieties of spondylolisthesis (McNab, 1977).

Transitional vertebra

A transitional vertebra is a fusion, in varying degree, of the transverse processes on one or both sides of two adjoining vertebrae, usually of L5 and S1. This in itself does not give rise to pain.

Tropism

Tropism is an asymmetry of the facet joints which leads to vertebral imbalance and therefore stress on structures.

Back pain may be a feature of the anomalies and deformities listed here, mainly because of the resulting stress on other tissues; on the other hand, the conditions may remain pain-free and often undetected throughout life.

This chapter has dealt with the bones of the back, the central edifice, the provider of rigidity; but the other important function of the back is movement. Bones cannot move without joints. The next chapter is about spinal motion.

REFERENCES

Arnoldi, C.C., Brodsky, A.E., Cauchoix, J.*et al.* (1976). Lumbar spinal stenosis and nerve root entrapment syndromes. *Clin. Orthop.*, **115**, 4–5.

Bogduk, N. and Twomey, L.T. (1991). *Clinical Anatomy of the Lumbar Spine*, 2nd ed., Churchill Livingstone.

In: Cash's Textbook of Orthopaedics and Rheumatology for Physiotherapists, (1992). Mosby Year Book Europe.

Crock, H.V. and Yoshizawa, H.(1976). The blood supply of the lumbar vertebral column. *Clin. Orthop.*, **115,** 6–21.

Darby, A.J. (1992). Bone and joint pathology, *In: Cash's Textbook of Orthopaedics and Rheumatology for Physiotherapists*, (Tidswell, M.E., ed.) 2nd ed., Mosby Year Book Europe.

Eisenstein, S. and Draycott, V. (1992). Spinal deformities. *In: Cash's Textbook of Orthopaedics and Rheumatology for Physiotherapists* (Tidswell, M.E., ed.), 2nd ed., Mosby Year Book Europe.

Evans, G.A. and Draycott, V. (1992). Childhood disorders of the hip and inequality of leg length. *In: Cash's Textbook of Orthopaedics and Rheumatology for Physiotherapists,* (Tidswell, M.E., ed.) 2nd ed., Mosby Year Book Europe.

Johnston, T.B. (1945) (ed.), *Gray's Anatomy*, Longmans, Green and Co.

Kapandji, I.A. (1974). *The Physiology of the Joints*, Vol. 3, The Trunk and the Vertebral Column, Churchill Livingstone.

Kirkaldy-Willis, W.H. and McIvor, G.W.D. (1976). Lumbar spinal stenosis, *Clin. Orthop.*, **115**, 2–3.

Kisner, C. and Colby, L.A. (1990). *Therapeutic Exercise. Foundations and Techniques*, 2nd ed., F.A. Davis Company, Philadelphia.

MacNab, I. (1977). *Backache*, Chapter 4, pp. 44–63, Williams and Wilkins.

Mourad, L.A. (1991). *Orthopedic Disorders*, Mosby Year Book Inc.

Porter, R.W. (1986). *Management of Back Pain*, Churchill Livingstone.

Taylor, J.R. and Twomey, L.T. (1987). The lumbar spine from infancy to old age. *In: Physical Therapy of the Low Back* (Twomey, L.T. and Taylor, J.R., eds.), Churchill Livingstone, USA.

Thomas, P.B.M. (1992). Fractures – Clinical. *In: Cash's Textbook of Orthopaedics and Rheumatology for Physiotherapists* (Tidswell, M.E., ed.), 2nd ed., Mosby Year Book Europe.

Twomey, L.T. and Taylor, J.R. (1987). Lumbar posture, movements and mechanics. *In: Physical Therapy of the Low Back* (Twomey, L.T. and Taylor, J.R., eds.), Churchill Livingstone, USA.

Twomey, L.T. (1989). Physical activity & ageing bones, *Patient Management Focus*, **August**, 27–34.

Wiltse, L. (1971). The effects of the common anomalies of the lumbar spine upon disc degeneration and low back pain, *Orthop. Clin. North Am.*, **2**(2), 569–582.

3. *The joints of the spine*

Joint mechanism

A joint is the meeting point between two bones. There may or may not be movement in the joint. For example, the hip joint has a vast range of movement, while at the other extreme, the joints between the bones of the skull have none.

Joints are classified by the type of material between them and they are of three kinds: synovial, cartilaginous and fibrous. Fibrous joints are immobile. The joints of the spine all move and they are of two types, synovial and cartilaginous.

Synovial joints

The bone ends or edges of a synovial joint are covered in a layer of **cartilage**, a smooth, resilient layer of dense connective tissue which varies in size and importance depending upon the stress expected of the joint; the knee cartilages play an essential role in cushioning the impact of weight bearing and are therefore different in size and shape from, for example, those of the finger joints.

Surrounding and enclosing the whole structure is a fibrous **capsule** which is lined by a **synovial membrane**. The synovial membrane secretes a thick **synovial fluid** into the joint (**3.1**). The synovial fluid keeps the

3.1

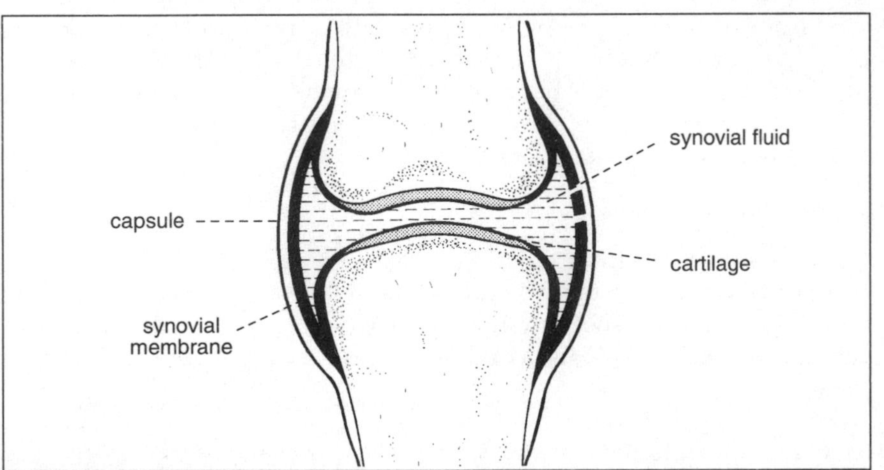

3.1 A basic synovial joint

joint friction-free, it bathes, lubricates and nourishes the cartilage, provides nutrients and oxygen for all the tissues and carries out phagocytic and other immunological functions within the joint (Mourad, 1991). Exercise stimulates its flow and the secretion tends to dry up with inactivity – another very important reason for continuing exercises into old age (Twomey, 1991). Injury causes the synovial fluid to increase, hence the swelling of any damaged joint.

The joint is surrounded at strategic places by tough, inelastic bands known as **ligaments**. These are sometimes incorporated into the capsule or they may cross the joint quite independently.

Ligaments have static and dynamic functions. Their static role is to prevent excessive movement and keep the joint compact. For this reason they are placed at positions of greatest stress to control undesirable movement and prevent dislocation. In normal movement the capsule and ligaments tighten and slacken around a joint depending on the accent of direction. Forced joint dislocation invariably damages these restraining tissues, sometimes causing tears or ruptures.

The dynamic aspect of ligaments is related to a proprioceptive function, a sensory feedback of muscle and joint information (Macleod *et al.*, 1987). Thus passive ligamentous stretching and reflex muscle control are closely linked and finely balanced (ibid).

It is important to understand ligamentous strains in the back, and the reaction of pain when they are put on stress. Try this experiment to test your own ligaments and feel their restraining influence. Grasp the tip of your index finger with your other hand and press the whole finger back as far as it will go, really hard. There will be a tight feeling at the bottom of the finger on the front where the skin and tissues are taut. The capsule and ligaments here are being stretched to their limit and are preventing excessive movement. Some people will be able to pull their fingers back much further than others because their ligaments allow greater range of joint movement. Acrobats are not 'double-jointed' – they merely have especially lax or long ligaments.

Cartilaginous joints

Cartilaginous joints are simpler. They have no capsule or synovial fluid, the cartilaginous substance being in the middle, attached to the bone ends on either side. The symphysis pubis, (See 2.3 p15), and the joint of the intervertebral disc, discussed below, are examples of cartilaginous joints.

All joints vary in the complexity and range of available movement. The middle joint of the finger, for example, has two active movements, flexion and extension. However, the shoulder joint can move in virtually any direction in any position, twisting and turning in different ways whether the arm is out at the side, above the head or behind the back. Its range of movement is huge, swinging through more than 200° from a position behind the back, forwards and up until it is above the head. The middle finger joint from its most bent position to the straight position moves through about 90–100°. Other joints fall somewhere between these two in the complexity of movement, many have considerably less range.

The vertebral joints

Each of the vertebral joints has a small range of movement, but their combined efforts throughout the spine create a large overall range. The mechanism is intricate but extremely effective.

There are three vertebral joints which form a triad. All three work together at all times: a large simple joint of the intervertebral disc and two small, more complicated zygapophyseal or facet joints.

The joints of the triad

The **intervertebral disc joint**
At every level, where vertebra meets vertebra, the intervertebral disc is placed like a tap-washer between the two vertebral bodies. It is a cushion or shock absorber transmitting the forces of weight-bearing down through the tough bones of the vertebral bodies. It is connected to the vertebral bodies above and below by a layer of cartilage (see intervertebral disc structure, p.34). The whole mechanism forms a cartilaginous joint which moves as the vertebrae rock to and fro, and from side to side.

The **zygapophyseal joints**
As the two vertebrae sit one on top of the other, the two zygapophyseal joints (the Z joints) are formed as the inferior articular processes of the top vertebra and the superior articular processes of the lower vertebra come together; they overlap and lock on to each other. Each forms a synovial joint, enclosed by a fibrous capsule with a layer of cartilage on the adjoining bony surfaces. The capsule is thickened by strong controlling ligaments. The Z joints are small but well designed to cope with the precise alteration of direction demanded of them in spinal movements. The angle and inclination of the joints change slightly from vertebra to vertebra so that the cervical spine Z joints are quite differently oriented from those of the lumbar spine. This enables the vertebrae to meet their different mobility requirements.

3.2

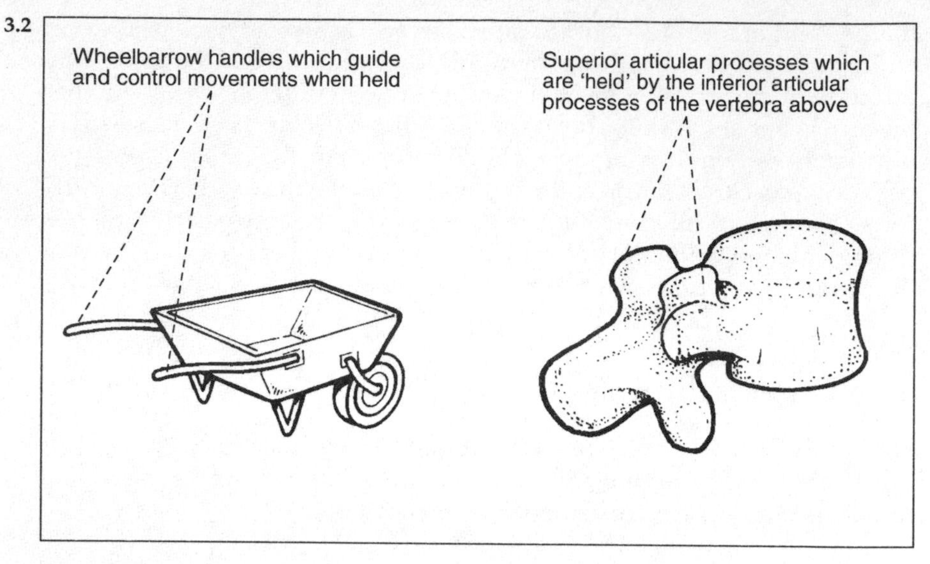

3.2 The triad 'wheelbarrow'

Mechanism of movement

The **mechanism of movement** of the triad is intricate and when examined in detail it varies from group to group in the different vertebrae, but the basic mechanism is similar throughout.

The disc joint is the major member of the triad, taking 80% of the weight-bearing force (Twomey and Taylor, 1987a), but the Z joints play an essential role of stabilisation, acting like the held handles of a wheelbarrow (**3.2**).

As the vertebral bodies rock backwards and forwards on each other during body movement, the Z joints to the rear stabilise and control any excessive tendency of the bodies to slide or glide on each other and to become unstable horizontally (Bogduk and Twomey, 1991). In their role as the 'handles of the wheelbarrow' the Z joints also restrict undue rotation and control excessive flexion in forward bending.

At each level the range of movement of the triad is very small but the overall large range of spinal movement is achieved by a spiral staircase effect: the bottom vertebra moves a few degrees while the next one up moves its few degrees in the same direction, so the effect is cumulative. This applies not only to the turning movement as in an actual spiral staircase, but also to bending forwards, sideways or backwards.

None of the three joints of the triad can function without having an effect on the others, as the triad formation is the essential element of spinal movement. A faulty performance in either can cause disruption in the function of

3.3

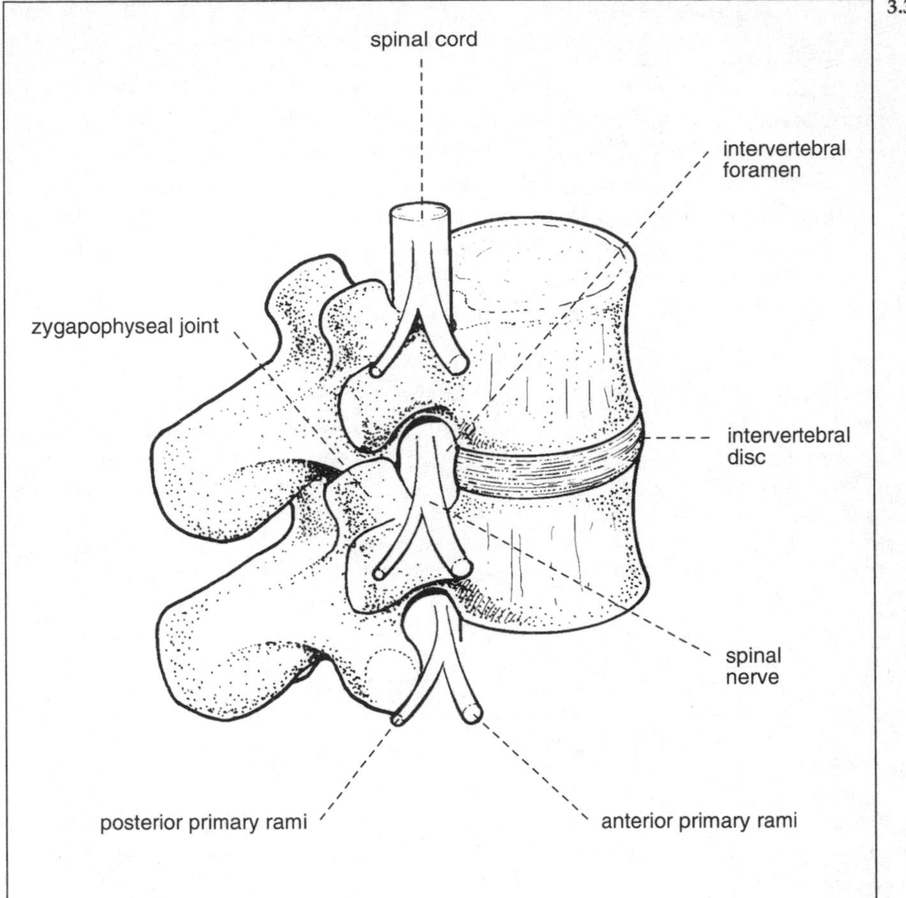

3.3 The motion segment

the other, so not only can a faulty disc cause strain on a Z joint but a faulty Z joint can equally create stress on a disc with resulting degenerative wear (Vernon-Roberts, 1992). The balanced interplay between disc and Z joint is crucial to perfect spinal co-ordination and function.

The motion segment

The two vertebrae and the structures around them form a motion segment of the spine, a duo that is repeated with slight variations of shape in each vertebral group throughout the spine. The coming together of the two vertebrae creates an opening on either side, the **intervertebral foramen** (IVF), an exit for any structures leaving the spinal canal (**3.3**). The spinal cord descends through the centre of the spinal canal, giving off a nerve on either side at regular intervals which exits through the IVF to supply the relevant body areas. Blood vessels also enter and exit through the IVF.

The intervertebral disc

A normal, healthy disc is a symmetrical kidney shape. In the average adult male, discs of the lumbar spine are about 1cm thick and the vertebral bodies above and below are about 2.5cm thick (Taylor and Twomey, 1987). Female sizes average 15% smaller. In order to perform its shock-absorbing function the disc needs to be malleable, adaptable to change of movement yet able to resume its form at rest. It must be strong enough to sustain weight, as load is transmitted from one vertebra to the next during all activities involving the spine. It must also remain uninjured by all this dynamic activity (Taylor and Twomey 1987). The intervertebral disc is composed of three parts:

- The nucleus pulposus in the centre.
- The annulus fibrosus surrounding the nucleus.
- Two vertebral end plates separating the whole structure from the vertebral bodies above and below (Markolf and Morris, 1974; Palastanga *et al.*, 1991) (**3.4**).

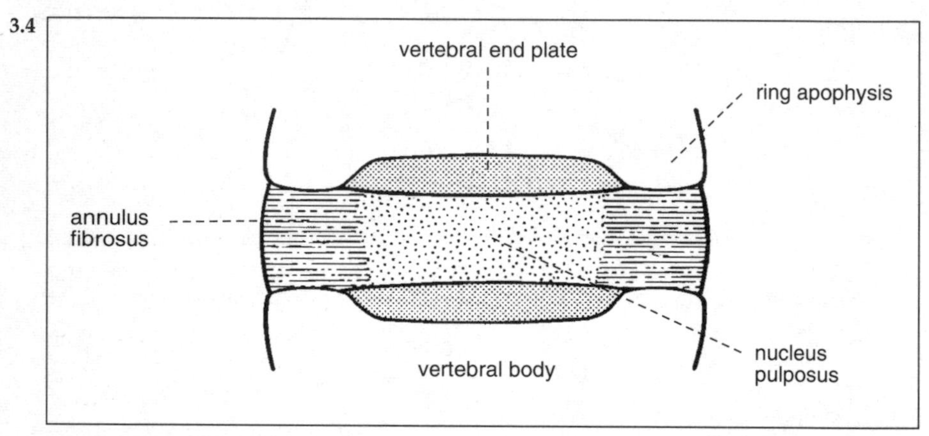

3.4 Cross-section of the disc and vertebral end plate

The nucleus pulposus is an oval-shaped gelatinous mass, a soft toothpaste-like substance which is made up of a certain amount of cartilage cells and collagenous fibres in a water-bound medium, 75–90% of its weight being fluid (Markolf and Morris, 1974). The nucleus is not quite like the jam in the middle of a doughnut as it is indistinctly separated from the surrounding annulus fibrosus, the two disc components having no obvious boundary between them. Because of its fluid nature the nucleus does not resist deformation in the way that rubber can, but is deformed under pressure like a water-filled balloon, the displaced pressure being transmitted in all directions towards the perimeter of the annulus (Bogduk and Twomey, 1991).

The annulus fibrosus is also made up of collagen fibres packed in a gel-like substance, with water amounting to 60–70% of its weight (Bogduk and

Twomey, 1991). The fibres are arranged in layers of concentric circles, like an onion. They surround the nucleus, with their fibres melding where they meet. The fibres of each layer run in obliquely opposite directions but as the layers are bound together by a cement-like substance the overall effect is of a lattice-like structure (Markolf and Morris, 1974). The anterior and lateral portions of the disc are thicker than the posterior part where the layers are more tightly packed (Bogduk and Twomey, 1991).

The vertebral end plate is a layer of cartilage covering the whole area of the vertebral body apart from the ring apophysis (see **2.6**, p. 18). It is attached to three-quarters of the disc surface, covering the nucleus entirely but leaving an area of annulus at the perimeter which is attached to the ring apophysis of the vertebral body (**3.4**).

Intervertebral disc mechanics

It is important to remember that the disc forms one of the anterior boundaries of the intervertebral foramen, and as the spinal nerve passes through the IVF it lies directly behind the disc (Palastanga *et al.*, 1991). The disc also forms part of the anterior wall of the spinal canal; a posterior bulge could therefore compromise the contents of the spinal canal as well as the spinal nerves (ibid).

The lattice construction of the annulus gives the disc its strength and ability to resist deformation from both pressure within the nucleus and load from the vertebral body. Although compressive forces descend through the vertebral bodies in all upright postures, straight compression has been found to be the least damaging force for the disc compared with sustained flexion and rotation (Markolf and Morris, 1974; Panjabi and White, 1980). As the vertebrae rock backwards and forwards in daily activity this characteristic is put to the test. Each change of direction squashes the disc, causing pressure within the nucleus to be dispersed into the fibres of the annulus and out towards the periphery. In flexion of the spine the disc is squashed in front, but pressure is exerted towards its stretched posterior annular boundary (McKenzie, 1981) (**3.5**). The opposite pressure is exerted in extension.

You can get some idea of the effect of intradiscal pressure if you imagine pressing on the centre of a balloon half-filled with water: the water in the balloon presses evenly towards the circumference all the way round. Now imagine altering the pressure of your hand in different directions: the water will push more towards one area of the circumference, stretching the perimeter. Add a twisting movement of your hand and the distortion on the balloon becomes considerable. If you now relate this to the spine, you can imagine the great stress exerted on the disc when the spine is flexed and the extra torsional strain that is added on twisting.

3.5

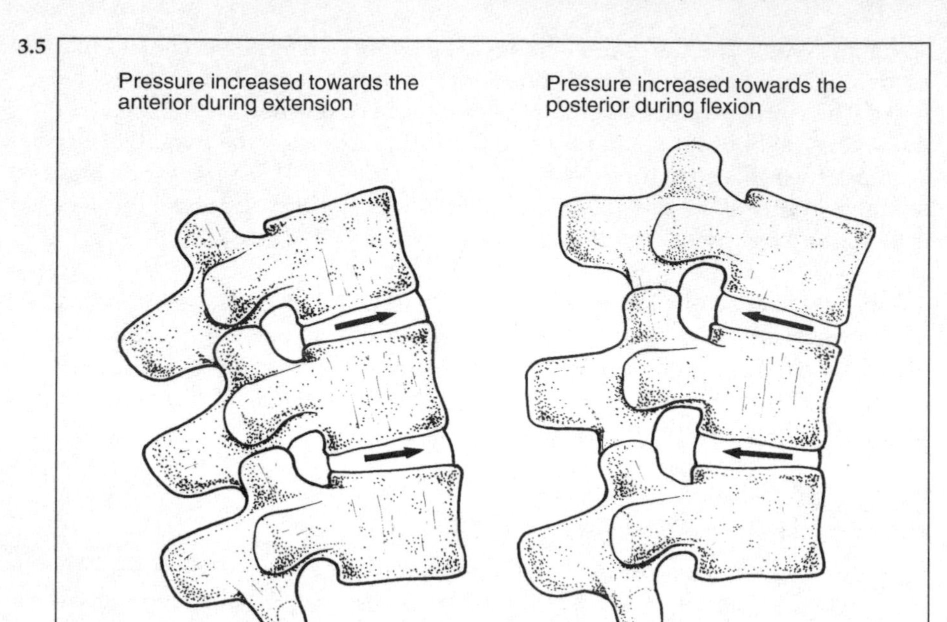

3.5 Movement of the nucleus under pressure

Torsional strain is one of the greatest causes of annular damage (Twomey and Taylor, 1987b). In flexion the potential towards torsional damage is increased as the rotational control exerted by the Z joints is less effective in this position (Panjabi and White, 1980).

In terms of back care, turning becomes an especially stressful and potentially harmful movement if performed in flexion, even more so when combined with holding an extra weight at the top of the twisting column. High-velocity torsional forces, such as whiplash injuries sustained in a rotated position, often result in tears of the annulus (Twomey and Taylor, 1987a).

Considerable research has been done on measurement of intradiscal pressures in order to validate theories regarding the effect of postural change on disc function. Intradiscal pressure varies according to posture (**3.6**); it is greater in standing than in lying, greater in sitting than in standing, greater in stooping than in a good lordotic position, increased in active flexion exercises and greatest of all in heavy lifting (Nachemson and Morris, 1964; Nachemson and Elfstrom, 1970; Andersson *et al.*, 1974; Andersson *et al.*, 1976). Merriam *et al.*, (1984) showed that degenerated discs behave in an inconsistent way which does not necessarily conform to the pressure changes of normal discs. All these facts provide a valid scientific backing to the theories of postural care (Nachemson, 1992).

3.6

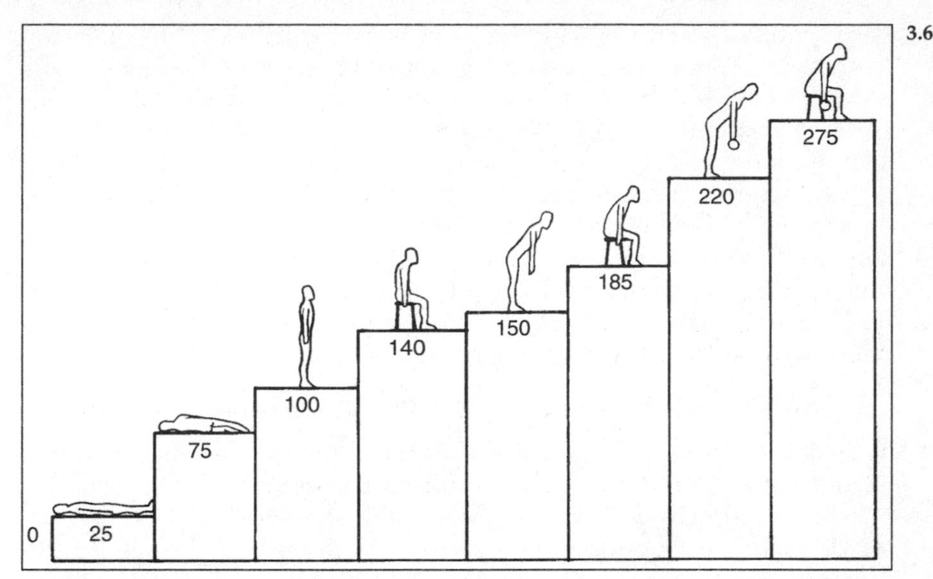

3.6 Relative increase and decrease in intradiscal pressure in different postures compared with the pressure in upright standing of 100%
(taken from Lumbar Intradiscal Pressure by Alf Nachemson, The Lumbar Spine and Back Pain, Ed. Malcolm I.V. Jayson, Churchill Livingstone 1987. With kind permission of the author and publishers)

Disc nutrition

Like all body tissue the disc needs nourishment. Nutrients are usually obtained from the blood, however, as the disc substance receives no major arterial branches it has to obtain nourishment from two sources:

- By **diffusion** from two arterial sources: a group of small arteries forming a fine network on the very periphery of the annulus and from a capillary plexus beneath the vertebral end plate (Urban *et al.*, 1977). Nutrients are passed through the tissues by the process of varying osmotic pressures.
- By fluid **absorption**. It is believed that there is a link between posture, fluid flow within the disc and nutrition (Adams and Hutton, 1983). Water content of the disc is variable and represents an equilibrium between two opposing pressures: a mechanical pressure which dehydrates the gel and rehydration pressure which causes the gel to absorb fluid from its surrounding tissues. Any change in the pressures put on the disc disturbs this equilibrium and fluid flows out until a new equilibrium is achieved. The fluid flow in and out of the disc alters its height and relates to its nutrition (Adams and Hutton, 1983).

Diurnal variation

During the night when the body is at rest, often lying curled up in flexed, unstressed postures, the discs tank up with fluid in preparation for the daily pounding. This is why the back feels particularly stiff on rising from sleep. The disc spaces are packed tight and there is literally less room for manoeuvre. We gain 1% of height during the night as a result (Adams and Hutton, 1983). During the day, through the pressures of activity in the upright posture, moisture is squeezed out of the disc and we lose height again. The greatest loss of fluid takes place in the first half hour of being upright, and in four hours fluid content is back to the daily average. In view of this the advisability of exercising immediately on rising from bed is questionable. A more sensible regime, especially for backs that are potentially at risk or recovering from pain, would be to delay exercise for at least half an hour, preferably longer, after rising.

In terms of **body movements** and **posture** three vital points emerge:

- Sustained loading of the discs in forward flexion (bending forwards under stress) produces fluid loss from the discs and loss of disc height which eventually deprives the disc of nourishment.
- Alternating periods of activity and rest with postural change tend to boost fluid exchange which increases nutrition.
- Flexion in the lying or unloaded position allows free flow of fluid through the annulus, sufficient to permit an increased fluid exchange to take place.

Three back care rules emerge from these three points:

- Avoid prolonged stooping
- Change position frequently
- Give the back a period of rest during each 24 hours, curled up in the horizontal position.

Any tissue deprived of nourishment will deteriorate, so apart from the actual mechanical stress of prolonged stooping, there is also a chemical or physiological reason for avoiding it and for advocating movement or exercise in quite simple forms.

Two movement rules emerge from this point:

- Maintaining one posture for long is bad, especially if that posture is a sustained or stressed flexion.
- Unstressed, controlled, full-range movement of the spine in all directions is good.

Innervation of the motion segment

There has been great controversy over the years regarding the innervation of the disc but recent findings have proved that there are abundant nerve endings in the outer fibres of the annulus (Bogduk and Twomey, 1991). There appears to be no nerve supply within the inner annular layers or in the nucleus. This distribution is highly significant in relation to the possible sources of back pain. The Z joints and other structures of the vertebral column, however, all have a liberal nerve supply.

The sacro-iliac joints

The sacro-iliac joint is technically not a joint of the vertebral column but as part of the base of the whole edifice it is important and is often part of the picture of low back pain.

The sacro-iliac is the joint between the sacrum and the ilium (see **2.3**, p. 15). The joint has minimal movement, mainly allowing for:

- A rotational 'give' as the weight of the spine tends to rock the sacrum between the hip bones.
- A slightly sideways glide as the ilium lifts during one-sided pelvic raise as in lifting one leg.
- A spreading-apart 'give' during pregnancy, accommodating the extra width needed in the pelvis.

Everyday movements of the joint occur during any weight transference from one leg to another, as in walking, climbing stairs or dancing; in turning to look behind while both feet remain stationary; or in stooping forwards while sitting.

Spinal ligaments

Ligaments are firm bands of fibrous tissue placed in and around joints.

3.7

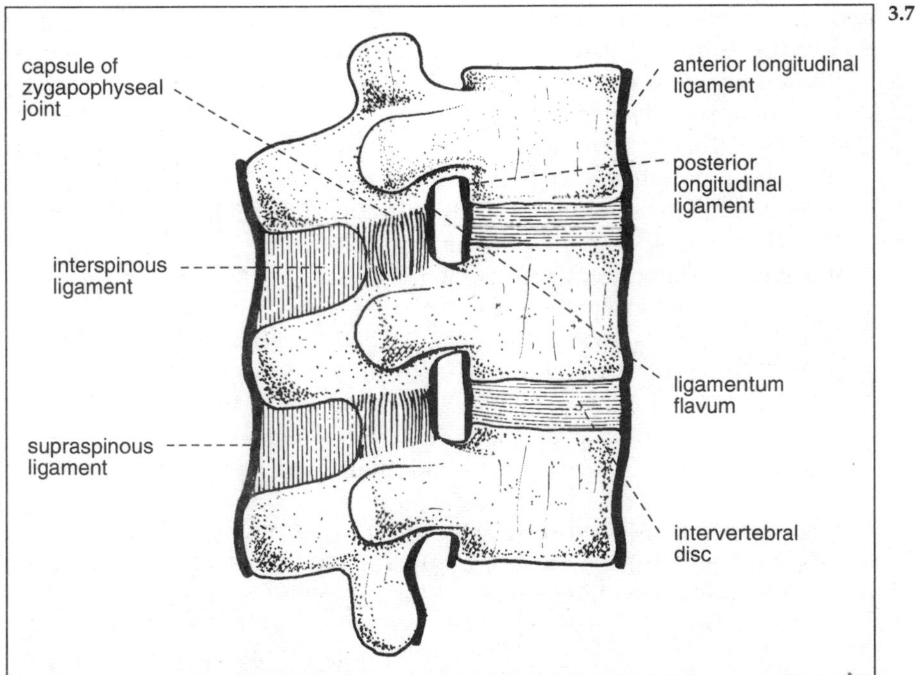

3.7 The major ligaments of the motion segment

They are like rubber bands in that they resist stretching but buckle when released. The various spines and protuberances of the vertebrae are connected to each other by numerous 'guy-ropes', each preventing undue movement, providing the whole edifice with a network of protection and stability. The main ligaments of the motion segment are shown in **3.7**.

The **ligaments of the anterior elements** of the vertebrae are the **anterior** and **posterior longitudinal ligaments** which run up and down the spine on the front and backs of the vertebral bodies and the disc. The annulus of the disc itself forms a ligamentous structure with its attachment to the ring apophysis of the vertebra above and below (Bogduk and Twomey, 1991) (see **3.4**). These ligaments regulate stretch and separation between two adjacent vertebral bodies.

The **ligaments of the posterior elements**, the **ligamentum flavum**, the **supraspinous** and **interspinous ligaments**, are related to functional control of spinal movements as they are stretched during flexion. The ligamentum flavum forms part of the capsular ligament of the Z joints and is the most elastic of all body ligaments (Panjabi and White, 1980). It lines the back of the spinal canal, where its elasticity maintains the smooth regular outline of the dural sac (the covering of the spinal cord) during movement (Taylor and Twomey, 1987a).

The ligaments of the lumbo-sacral area are the ilio-lumbar ligaments and those of the sacro-iliac joint:

- The **ilio-lumbar ligaments** join the transverse processes of L5 to the ilium, forming a strong bond between them and acting to prevent L5 slipping forwards on the sacrum.
- **The sacro-iliac** is surrounded on both sides of the joint by a strong mass of ligamentous structures which are normally firm and tight. However, during pregnancy hormonal changes induce a laxity in the ligaments of the sacro-iliac and of the lumbar spine allowing for greater range of movement. This creates a vulnerability to stress which can in turn lead to pain. A similar situation arises during menstruation with the same tendency towards sacral and lumbar pain. Sacro-iliac pain during pregnancy can be successfully treated with physiotherapy but in most cases it is relieved immediately after delivery. There may be remaining uncertainty in the joint for at least four months post-partum requiring a great deal of back care, especially as new mothers bend and lift more often.

A considerable amount of pain in the area of the sacro-iliac which is ascribed to the joint is however often misdiagnosed and is, instead, a referred pain from the lumbar spine.

The blood supply of the motion segment

The motion segment receives a liberal blood supply from the lumbar arteries and veins. Apart from the intervertebral discs, which have only an anastomosis of small blood vessels on the outer surface of the annulus fibrosus, a network of blood vessels enmeshes the rest of the whole motion segment providing nutrients to the vertebral body, the Z joints and all surrounding structures, including branches that enter the intervertebral foramen providing a blood supply for the spinal cord and structures within the spinal canals. (Bogduk and Twomey, 1991).

REFERENCES

Adams, M.A. and Hutton, W.C. (1983). The effect of posture on the fluid content of the lumbar intervertebral discs, *Spine*, **8**(6), 665–671.

Andersson, B.J.B., Ortengren, R., Nachemson, A. *et al.* (1974). Lumbar disc pressure and myoelectric back muscle activity during sitting, *Scand. J. Rehabil. Med.*, **6**, 104.

Andersson, B.J.B., Ortengren, R. and Nachemson, A. (1976). Quantitative studies of back loads in lifting, *Spine*, **1**(3), 178.

Bogduk, N. and Twomey, L.T. (1991). *Clinical Anatomy of the Lumbar Spine*, Churchill Livingstone.

Macleod, D., Maughan, R., Nimmo, M., Reilly, T. and Williams, C. (1987). *Exercise, Benefits, Limits and Adaptations*, E. & F.N. Spon Ltd.

Markolf, K.L. and Morris, J.M. (1974). The structural components of the intervertebral disc, *J. Bone Joint Surg.*, **56A**(4), 675–687.

McKenzie, R. (1981). *The Lumbar Spine: Mechanical Diagnosis and Therapy*, Spinal Publications.

Merriam, W.F., Quinnell, R.C., Stockdale, H.R. *et al.* (1984). The effect of postural changes on the inferred pressures within the nucleus pulposus during lumbar discography, *Spine*, **9**(4), 406.

Mourad, L.A. (1991). *Orthopedic Disorders.*, Mosby Year Book.

Nachemson, A. (1992). Lumbar mechanisms as revealed by lumbar intradiscal pressure measurements. *In: The Lumbar Spine and Back Pain* (Jayson, M.I.V. ed.), 4th ed, Churchill Livingstone.

Nachemson, A. and Elfstrom, G. (1970). Intravital dynamic pressure measurements in lumbar discs. *Scand. J. Rehab. Med., suppl* **1**(1).

Nachemson, A. and Morris J.M. (1964). In vivo measurements of intradiscal pressure, *J. Bone Joint Surg.*, **46A**(5), 1077–1092.

Palastanga, N., Field, D. and Soames, R. (1991). *Anatomy and Human Movement*, Heinemann Medical Books.

Panjabi, M.M. and White, A.A. (1980). Basic biomechanics of the spine. *Neurosurgery*, **7**(1), 76–93.

Taylor, J.R. and Twomey, L.T. (1987). The lumbar spine from infancy to old age *In: Physical Therapy of the Low Back* (Twomey, L.T. and Taylor, J.R. eds), Churchill Livingstone, USA.

Twomey, L.T. (1991). Musculoskeletal physiotherapy: the age of reason, *Proceedings of the 11th Congress of the World Confederation for Physical Therapy*, **1**, 343–347.

Twomey, L.T. and Taylor, J.R. (1987a). Lumbar posture, movement, and mechanics. *In: Physical Therapy of the Low Back* (Twomey, L.T. and Taylor, J.R. eds.), Churchill Livingstone, USA.

Twomey, L.T. and Taylor, J.R. (1987b). Age changes in the lumbar vertebrae & intervertebral discs, *Clin. Orthop.*, **224**(November), 97–103.

Urban, J.P.G., Holm, S., Markoudas, A. and Nachemson, A. (1977). Nutrition of the Intervertebral Disc. *Clin. Orthop.*, **129** (Nov-Dec), 101–114.

Vernon-Roberts, B. (1992). Age-related and degenerative pathology of the intervertebral discs and apophyseal joints, *In: The Lumbar Spine and Back Pain* (Jayson, M.I.V. ed.), 4th ed, Churchill Livingstone.

4. Disorders of the motion segment

Misconceptions

Back pain has been discussed throughout history with reasons given for its onset ranging from punishment from heaven for sins committed, to sitting in a draught, to 'just a muscle strain'. In recent years our understanding of the mechanisms involved has become more scientific in every way, but the precise cause of pain is still often obscure, mainly because of the number and complexity of structures which can be implicated.

However, in the search for knowledge certain myths and old wives' tales have been invalidated. One of the more controversial claims used by some manipulators is that a bone in the back is 'out', waiting to be dramatically 'put back', thus reducing or curing all pain. This idea needs to be firmly refuted. A spinal dislocation would only occur after a major accident such as a bad road traffic accident, an aeroplane crash, or a twisting fall, the results of dislocation being extremely severe.

Perhaps the error of diagnosis results from a misunderstanding of the postural deviation evoked by muscle spasm. Severe pain can elicit a protective reaction in the muscles of the back, causing them to contract involuntarily in an attempt to avoid pain by preventing movement. The contraction can be sufficiently strong to pull the spine into an artificial scoliosis, deviating the whole line of vertebrae to one side, sometimes producing a kink at one particular vertebra. The spasm can also cause one vertebra to rotate slightly, making the spinous process appear out of alignment with its neighbours. Depending on the cause of pain, manipulation could have a curative effect, possibly by affecting a joint – but not because a bone has been 'put back' in place.

The second myth in need of clarification is the one concerning draughts. If we are submitted to cold severe enough to cause an appreciable drop in body temperature, our circulation will be affected with resulting alteration in the tissues. A draught wafting over the surface anatomy of the body is another matter. If pain is the aftermath of being in a draught it is not because of the breeze but as a consequence of our own muscular tension, hunching the shoulders or stiffening the back, in an attempt to protect ourselves against discomfort.

The third and perhaps the most common misconception met with every day is the claim that pain can be caused by a 'slipped disc'. The diagnosis seems to be made by all and sundry during any acute attack of back pain, especially if spinal X-rays have shown a narrowing or irregularity in the disc space. X-rays show only bone, the condition of the bone, the spinal alignment and the shape of the disc space between the vertebral bodies. If there is alteration in the disc space it is probable that the disc is worn or even destroyed in some way which may or may not be relevant to the particular pain. Discs narrow, bulge, herniate, degenerate, disrupt, become deranged and suffer degradation but they *do not slip*.

Disorders and ageing of the intervertebral disc and the vertebral end plate

A young healthy intervertebral disc is strong, resilient and elastic, able to accept both deformation – followed by return to its former shape, and dehydration – followed by its own speedy process of rehydration. However, throughout the course of any normal active life, even discounting the more noticeable traumatic events, the disc suffers constant abuse from all angles.

Stressed forces in flexion, extension and rotation repeatedly pressurise the nucleus into the annulus, eventually giving rise to areas of wear in the inner annulus (Markolf and Morris, 1974; Panjabi and White, 1980). These lines of wear will not themselves generate pain unless they spread in the form of radial fissures into the outer, innervated annular layers. Any disc lesion can remain undetected providing:

- The disturbance remains within the inner annulus.
- The outer layers do not become involved.
- The disc in no way compromises the sensitive structures within the spinal canal or IVF.

The potential for damage lies in the disc's reaction to progressive deformation, that is loss of fluid content. As described in Chapter 3 (p. 35), deformation occurs in the upright position both in sustained extension and in sustained flexion (as opposed to relaxed, unloaded flexion in lying), though sustained flexion is a far more common posture in daily activity.

Sustained flexion not only squeezes fluid out from the discs, the articular cartilage of the Z joints and the spinal ligaments but it distorts and reshapes the discs and other soft tissues by redistributing the remaining fluid in them (Twomey *et al.*, 1988). The longer the static hold, the longer the recovery period, and the greater the potential disc damage.

Repetitive high-velocity forces, especially when associated with rotation, can initiate annular tears or extend lines of wear already present (Adams and Hutton, 1985). Of the three most potentially damaging forces of compression, torsion and flexion, torsion and flexion are more likely to cause failure of the annulus into a posterior protrusion; compression is more likely to affect the vertebral end plate and vertebral body (Hickey and Hukins, 1980).

Wear and tear together with trauma thus lead to a variety of changes within the disc. Some of those changes are described below.

Disc derangement

Disc derangement is a mechanical disturbance of the disc which can occur in stages or as a result of sudden trauma (Adams and Hutton, 1982). It occurs more readily in younger people, the elderly being saved by their stiffer, less fluid nuclei and less deformable discs.The process of disc derangement from normal healthy disc, through wear and continued pressure to herniation was described as long ago as 1934 by Mixter and Barr and by others since including McKenzie (1981) and Adams and Hutton (1985) (see **4.1–4.4**).

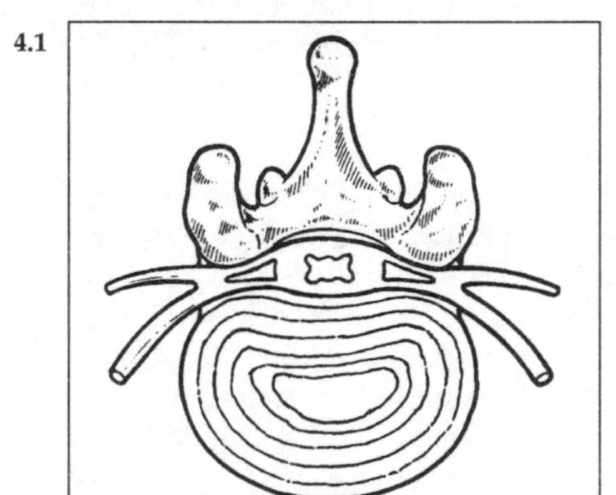

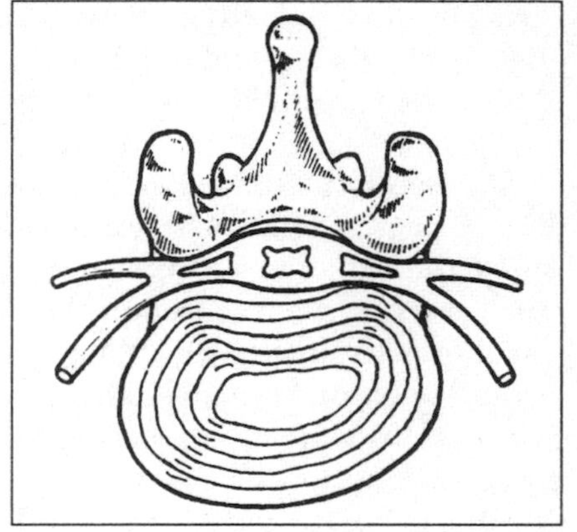

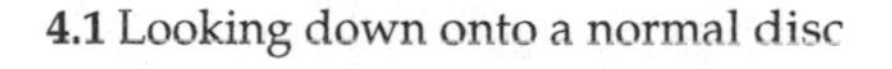

4.1 Looking down onto a normal disc

4.2 The disc showing signs of wear

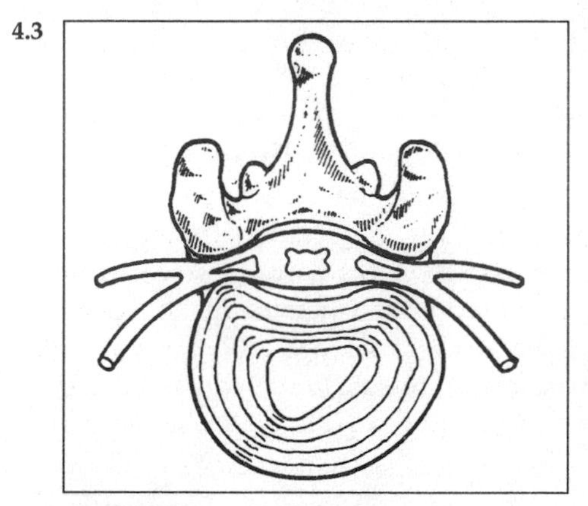

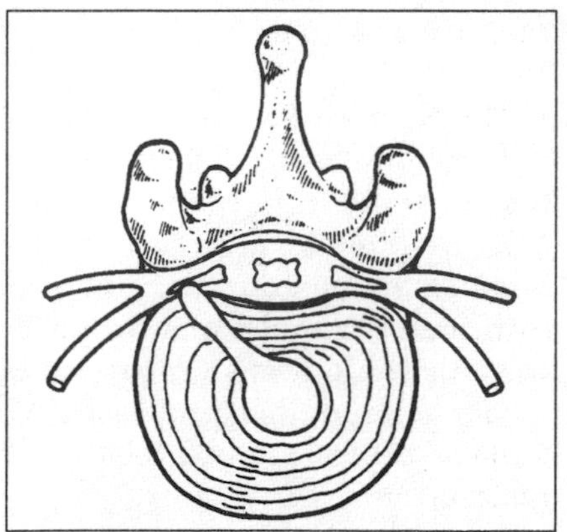

4.3 A line of wear starts to become a disc bulge

4.4 A herniating disc with extrusion onto the nerve root

Prolonged abuse of sustained and repetitive postures (Hickey and Hukins, 1980) causes the disc to develop the lines of wear described above (**4.2**). The lines extend into radial fissures or tears of the inner annulus, becoming an internal disc derangement. Pain will be experienced only if the fissures extend into the perimeter of the disc, when treatment may be necessary. Recovery can be spontaneous at this stage and can be complete if full movement is regained with back care executed meticulously. However, with repetitive abuse or poor recovery, the weak lines of stress in the annulus cannot withstand the continued pressure, the annulus bulges, just as an old balloon thins and bulges, and becomes a protruding disc (**4.3**). Areas of weakness can occur at any point on the perimeter but the most common site is at the back of the disc, towards either side, the area most pressurised by forward bending in rotation (see **3.5**, p. 36).

Unfortunately, to the rear of the disc lie all the pain-sensitive structures of the spinal canal (see Chapter 6). Pressure or irritation of these structures can cause symptoms of pain in the back or pain, pins and needles (paraesthesia) and numbness (anaesthesia) down the leg. Again, this stage can recover with the bulge retracting and the tissues healing.

The result of a bulge that has not resolved and can stand the strain no longer is shown in (**4.4**). Any sudden, possibly small movement can cause the bulge to weaken and become a disc herniation. Part of the nuclear pulp bursts through the annulus and extrudes into the spinal canal or area of the IVF (Adams and Hutton, 1985). If the herniation is gross, the extruded material may have to be removed from the surrounding areas by operative procedure but it is possible for it to be absorbed naturally and for the disc to heal, such are the self-sealing properties of the disc (Markolf and Morris, 1974).

Stages **4.1–4.3** can occur at any age but stage **4.4** is unlikely to occur in the older disc as the nucleus is less fluid (see ageing of the disc below).

This form of herniation as an anatomic concept, accepted for a long time, is now being challenged as representing only one facet of the true biological model (Lipson, 1988). It has been found that protrusion or prolapse need not involve the nucleus pulposus but can occur with degeneration of the annulus with the annular fibres protruding or prolapsing into the vertebral canal or, yet more strangely, protruding inwards towards the nucleus (Yasuma *et al.*, 1988; Yasuma *et al.*, 1990). Lipson (1988) believes that proliferation of annular tissue may well instigate annular protrusion or prolapse which may not be related to any traumatic event.

The clinical picture which accompanies any gradual mechanical derangement is one of repetitive incidents of low back pain with or without referral of pain into the buttocks and legs, usually increasing in severity and length of time for recovery. Depending on the amount of soft tissue involvement the pain can be constant but more often it is relieved by certain positions or movements and aggravated by others. This is an occasion when the analysis of pain and the understanding of the process of injury and healing can make all the difference between success or failure of recovery.

The diagnosis of disc protrusion or prolapse can only be made accurately by a myelogram, discography, computerised tomography (CT) scan or magnetic resonance imaging (MRI). Normal radiography will show nothing conclusive. Many cadavers have been examined showing disc bulges in spines that have been known to be pain-free, so once again pathological change does not necessarily lead to pain.

Internal disc disruption

Trauma to a disc from heavy lifting or from the high-speed application of force, for example the compressive thrust of a heavy fall, can damage the disc or fracture the vertebral end plate. In the disc itself trauma can result in nuclear degradation whereby a chemical destruction of the nucleus takes place. Inflammatory nuclear material may then advance along radial fissures causing erosion of the annulus (Bogduk and Twomey, 1991). The result can be the production of noxious substances which may either drain into the spinal canal, irritating nerves in the vicinity, or pass into the vertebral body through the capillaries of the vertebral end plate (Crock, 1986).

Crock has put forward an hypothesis suggesting that the irritating substances that enter the circulation via the vertebral end plate or that drain into the spinal canal can set up an auto-immune reaction which would present the following syndrome:

- Intractable pain, increased considerably on movement.
- Leg pain.
- Loss of energy.
- Marked weight loss.
- Profound depression.

Patients with this syndrome would have normal X-rays, normal myelogram, normal spinal CT scans and normal neurological findings. The only accurate diagnosis could be made through discography (Crock, 1986). Reviewing the anatomy and pathophysiology of whiplash, Bogduk (1986) describes many similar symptoms relating to the cervical spine and upper limbs.

Disc degeneration

Disc degeneration is often ill-defined but it is best described as a consequence of wear and tear or injury, not an inevitable part of the process of ageing (Twomey, 1991). The effect can be comparable with the mechanical early changes described in 'disc derangement' or it can be a nuclear degradation, causing the nucleus to discolour and change consistency (Vernon-Roberts, 1992). There is inevitably loss of disc height. The loss of height can compromise the mechanics of the whole motion segment causing increasing wear on the Z joints and the surrounding soft tissue.

Disc narrowing

Disc narrowing is noticeable on X-ray of a number of patients with back pain. It is believed to result from either loss of disc material from herniation or from disc dehydration or disc degradation, as mentioned above. Disc narrowing occurs mainly at specific discs which bear the greatest strain of weight bearing, especially between L5 and S1; it is rarely universal throughout all the discs of one spine. Research recorded by Twomey and Taylor (1987 and 1991) and Bogduk and Twomey (1991) has shown that although disc narrowing is seen mostly in elderly people, possibly because they are the ones who have more frequent X-rays, it is by no means a phenomenon of ageing.

Ageing of the disc

The fundamental age changes in the disc are biochemical. The collagen content of both the nucleus and annulus become greater but there is less distinction between the two areas. The water-binding capacity of the disc decreases, causing the disc to be dehydrated and less elastic (Bogduk and Twomey, 1991). The speed of deformation becomes slower, but the amount of deformation is greater and the recovery time longer (Twomey *et al.*, 1988). In this way ageing affects the flexibility of the disc and thus the mobility of the spine.

Contrary to some belief the discs tend to enlarge with age, ballooning centrally into the body of the adjacent vertebrae which, because of the age-related loss of bone density, become concave at the junction with the vertebral end plate (Twomey and Taylor, 1991). In fact the loss of elderly stature is not due to loss of disc height but rather more to the loss in height of the vertebral body (Twomey and Taylor, 1991).

Disorders of the vertebral end plate

The vertebral end plate is the weakest part of the motion segment. Fractures can occur in compression and torsional injuries such as a fall from a height, explosion blasts, road accidents and rugby-type injuries. Fortunately perhaps, the vertebral end plate has no nerve supply and so injuries need not be symptomatic. They can heal with no ill effects but changes may result if healing is incomplete (Bogduk and Twomey, 1991). End plate fractures can evoke an inflammatory repair response that can extend beyond the fracture site and invade the nucleus leading to nuclear degradation and protrusion of the nucleus into the vertebral body. Nuclear extrusion into the vertebral body can form Schmorl's nodes (see p. 53).

The cartilage of the vertebral end plate thins with age, and when bowing into the concavity of the vertebral body occurs, tiny microfractures can appear in the cartilage. These, like many structural changes may never give pain and may never be known about.

Disorders of the zygapophyseal joints

In their stabilising role as part of the vertebral joint triad, the Z joints are under constant stress. Not only do they break any tendency of the vertebral bodies to slide, they also control all movements. To return to the metaphor of the wheelbarrow – if something is amiss with the wheel, causing the barrow to tip to one side, the hand on that side has to do a lot more work to control the steady movement of the whole barrow.

For many years the disc was considered to be the main source of back pain but later investigations of the Z joints revealed that they too could be the culprits: the term 'facet syndrome' was coined (Mooney and Robertson, 1976). The Z joints have a liberal nerve supply and pain can originate from:

- A capsular reaction to trauma.
- Incompetence of the joint due to stress.
- Degenerative conditions of the joint.

In any clinical situation now therapists are very aware of the important role dysfunction of these joints plays in the search for the source of pain.

Age changes in the Z joints

As the Z joints are under considerable stress throughout life most of the changes that occur are those related to wear and tear.The cartilage of the Z joints, damaged by sustained loading, thickens in places and thins in others, depending on the angles of stress. Splits can appear in the cartilage substance. The capsule thickens and becomes less elastic.

Changes can occur at the joint margins where **osteophytes** may develop. These beak-like outgrowths of bone are believed to develop as a protective mechanism at points of stress, for example near ligamentous attachments. The osteophytes of the Z joints are accompanied by enlarged synovial fat pads which form cushions between the osteophytes and the inferior articular process (Taylor and Twomey, 1986; Vernon-Roberts, 1992).

General vertebral disorders

Certain disorders of the spine have, in the past, been considered to be 'diseases', but they are now accepted as degenerative changes which may or may not be part of the pain syndrome presented.

Three of the most commonly encountered terms are 'spondylosis', 'arthritis' and 'degenerative joint disease'. They are three terms which are, unfortunately, often thrown at patients as a diagnosis which seems to insinuate: 'you have a whole lot of arthritic and degenerative changes in your spine, nothing can be done about it and you must expect to have pain'. The effect on patients is often appalling, partly because the word 'arthritis' in itself conjures up pictures of total disability with the use of aids and wheelchairs and partly because 'there is no cure'.

Arthritis

The word 'arthritis' is derived from the Greek *arthron* meaning 'joint'. So arthritis means 'inflammation of a joint', which does not say a great deal. As there are several different forms of arthritis it is essential to explain to patients that in order to relate the term to any bodily condition, another qualifying word must be used, for example, 'osteo-arthritis' or 'rheumatoid-arthritis'. These are the two which are most frequently confused, the confusion not surprisingly leading to alarm.

Rheumatoid Arthritis (RA) is a chronic, systemic, autoimmune inflammatory disease of the connective tissues of the body (Mourad, 1991). It is one which involves the body as a whole. The exact aetiology is unknown but current hypotheses suggest that both genetic and microbiological factors may be important; there is some familial element (Grennan and Jayson, 1984).

- Symptoms usually start in the small joints of the hand or feet but any joint can be affected as the disease progresses, including the spine.
- The more severe the condition, the more widespread its effect.
- The membrane lining the joint capsule becomes inflamed, causing the joint to be red, swollen, stiff and extremely painful; the skin can appear quite shiny.
- The muscles around the joint become weak and wasted.
- Bone erosion begins at the joint margins, then with continued bone and cartilage destruction the joints become irreversibly deformed (ibid).
- The disease affects adults mainly between the ages of 20 and 55, women rather more than men, but it also appears in children when it known as Still's disease. There is often a feeling of general malaise and lassitude, with weight loss and low grade pyrexia. The disease has periods of remission when it is quiescent, followed by periods of severity, or it can remit spontaneously (Grennan and Jayson, 1984; Butler and Kerr, 1992).

- Diagnosis is made by blood test, giving a raised erythrocyte sedimentation rate (ESR). X-rays show the changes in the joint cartilage and bone ends (Mourad, 1991; Butler and Kerr, 1992).
- Treatment is mainly medical in the form of steroidal drugs but physiotherapy can help to reduce pain and maintain joint movement (Butler and Kerr, 1992).

Osteoarthritis (OA) is not a systemic disease – it can be defined as a joint's inadequacy to meet the mechanical stress placed upon it, or as wear and tear in any specific joint, but there is considerable clinical and pathological evidence of an inflammatory component of the condition (Harkness *et al.*, 1984). It can also be the result of abnormal metabolic, physiological or pathological factors (Ward *et al.*, 1992).

- The joints most frequently affected are those most under stress, usually the large, weight-bearing joints of the hip and knee or the small joints at the base of the thumb.
- OA can occur in one joint or several joints (but unrelated to each other) and the condition in itself is not progressive.
- OA is a degenerative condition involving the cartilage and bone ends in joints and as such can be present without pain. Under stress, however, the joints can become inflamed and swollen; pain-sensitive structures in the area will then be affected.
- The muscles around an OA joint only weaken through lack of use.
- Joints can be deformed if the condition becomes gross.
- Most people over the age of 30 develop OA somewhere and the majority of people have OA of the spine by the time they reach old age.
- Diagnosis is made by X-ray which shows degeneration of the cartilage, joint space loss, sclerosis of bone and osteophytes. Medication helps only if there is an inflammatory reaction but physiotherapy can help with mobilisation of the joint together with strengthening exercises for the muscles of support..
- Treatment is by prevention rather than cure. Once degeneration takes place the clock cannot be put back, but the symptoms of stiffness, swelling, inflammation or pain, if present, can be alleviated to almost nil providing the joint degeneration is not too great and that it is cared for in the right way.

People's reaction to new stiffness is generally to avoid movement. For example, if we find that we cannot turn our head on reversing the car or crossing the road, our common response is anxiety and the restriction of all head movements. The opposite should be the case – at the first sign of stiffness or slight pain, providing there has been no immediate trauma, a joint should be encouraged to achieve its full range of movement by persistent, gentle nudging into the stiffness. Stress that may have triggered the problem should be avoided, the muscles around the joint strengthened with exercises and the joint used as normally as possible with minimum weight-bearing stress. Maintenance of joint movement range is one of the most important safeguards against painful OA. Thousands of people live and die with pain-free OA, knowing nothing of its existence.

Spondylosis, osteoarthrosis and degenerative joint disease

These are not 'diseases', but degenerative conditions of the vertebral column.

Spondylosis usually describes disc narrowing and osteophytic formation along the junction of the vertebral bodies and their intervertebral discs (Bogduk and Twomey, 1991; Vernon-Roberts, 1992). Osteo-phytes are beak-like outgrowths composed of dense bone, more compact and stronger than the vertebral bodies which are often osteoporotic. They can be viewed as a reactive and adaptive change that seeks to compensate for biomechanical failure (Bogduk and Twomey, 1991). As the vertebrae become more osteoporotic with age, the osteophytes become larger and more numerous. They can grow from the vertebral bodies until they meet, forming the vertebrae into a pillar-like shape which acts as a support against increased pressure. By growing onto the disc surfaces of the vertebral bodies, they can double the size of the original body, thus reducing pressure by dispersing it (Nathan and Israel, 1962). Whether or not osteophytes cause pain depends entirely upon whether they compromise soft tissue in the area.

Osteoarthrosis and **degenerative joint disease** are extensive osteoarthritis of the Z joints as a result of constant stress throughout life.

In all degenerative disorders adaptive changes occur when the stressed tissues are capable of remodelling and opposing the applied stress, but if the stresses are severe or repetitive, destructive features may develop (Bogduk and Twomey, 1991). The problem of all degenerative conditions is that the joint is no longer able to withstand stress. If a 60-year-old and a 10-year-old both trip over a mat, the 60-year-old is likely to have pain afterwards while the youngster escapes with no aftermath.

Spondylitis

Spondylitis is a degenerative inflammation of the joints of the spine. **Ankylosing spondylitis** is an inflammatory disease of the spinal column in which ossification of the spinal ligaments and bony ankylosis occurs. It is a progressive disease of the spine and larger joints, such as the hips and shoulders, which is self-limiting but may result in complete fusion of the spinal column, giving rise to the term 'bamboo spine' because on X-ray the spine looks like a bamboo cane (Mourad, 1991). Morning backache with sacro-iliac pain are early symptoms. Treatment consists of non-steroidal anti-inflammatory drugs and a rigorous exercise routine with diligent postural correction (Dixey and Kerr, 1992).

Schmorl's nodes

Although, as mentioned earlier, **Schmorl's nodes** can develop in an older spine as a result of fracture of the vertebral end plate, they are more commonly found in adolescent spines where the developing cartilage end plates leave weak areas. Protrusion of nuclear material into the vertebral bodies can result. They can be asymptomatic. (Taylor and Twomey, 1987; Vernon-Roberts, 1992).

Scheuermann's disease

Scheuermann's osteochondritis occurs in adolescence and is a common cause of thoracic kyphosis. Diagnosis is made on lateral radiographs of the spine. Large anterior Schmorl's nodes are often seen and are sometimes associated with anterior vertebral body collapse leading to a wedge shaped vertebra. The disorder tends to be more painful in the lumbar or dorso-lumbar spine. The cause is unknown but it is thought to be associated with some weakness of the vertebral end plate (Taylor and Twomey, 1987; Galasko, 1992).

There is a relationship between lumbar Scheuermann's disease and hard physical labour in teenagers and it occurs more commonly in young athletes (Galasko, 1992). Pain usually responds to rest and, if necessary, immobilisation or bracing (ibid).

The clinical picture

Most disorders of the vertebral column listed above can be present without pain or they can be a part of the pain picture of a patient who requires help. Many of the age-related changes could have been present for years, causing no problems, yet they could now be compromised by trauma or stiffness or inflammation for some reason.

X-rays may show osteophytes at certain levels, disc narrowing at another and yet on examination the pain may be coming from quite another source, possibly from a more healthy-looking motion segment under stress because it is taking greater strain. Diagnosis is often unrelated to any of these specific conditions, but rather to a stress or strain imposed upon the vertebral structures, whether showing degeneration or not. You have to think in terms of function and loss of function both in relation to your own pain and in relation to other people's.

Painful conditions of the back can arise from a disturbance of any pain-sensitive structure of the motion segment including the muscles attached to or passing over it. Any classification presents a difficulty because there is rarely one source of pain or one name to give that pain (Bogduk, 1992).

Postural pain

Pain can arise from poor postural habits where joints are placed under long-term stress or stress formed repetitive nagging movements.

Sustained stress. The experiment (see Chapter 3, p. 30) of pulling your finger back until you felt pain was an example of sustained stress. Sustained stress or strain can occur in flexion or extension. It results from any poor posture where the joints sag into the end of their range, hanging the weight into stretched soft tissue and remaining in that position for hours. The stress may not be sufficiently great to cause pain for some time until the cumulative effect builds up.

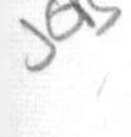

- **Sustained flexion** stress occurs in all activities which take place in a sitting or stooping posture. It is a potential source for the troubles discussed in this chapter.
- **Sustained extension** stress is rarer because extension is used less in occupations, but it does occur in prolonged standing, especially in exaggerated lordotic postures (see Chapter 11, p. 123). The stress is mainly on the Z joints as they are forced into extreme extension; in severe cases the inferior facets can become impacted upon the lamina. The condition, in the elderly, can be further extended into one of 'kissing spines' when the spinous processes actually meet each other (Taylor and Twomey, 1987).

Repetitive stress is movement without respite or change. It entails bending a little way forwards and then a little way up, over and over, without ever really straightening. All the structures that control the movement become fatigued.

- **Repetitive flexion** is the most common activity of life. It is part of all manual work, most household work, all nursing and medical procedures, jobs involving the care of small children, and many postures used in manufacturing.
- **Repetitive extension** postures that do not also contain trauma are more rare; painting a ceiling is one of the few examples but even this is saved by the need to change position and get more paint!

The nagging abuse of these postures can affect ligaments, joint cartilages, joint capsules and the discs not only from stress but also from the lack of nutrition of the joint provided by full-range active movement (Taylor and Twomey, 1987). Static postures actually initiate age change and degeneration.

Symptoms are usually intermittent in nature, occurring during the performance of activities which keep the lumbar spine in a relatively static position – as in vacuuming – or while maintaining end-of-range positions for long periods – as in stooping over a bed. (McKenzie, 1981). Activity usually eases the pain.

Joint dysfunction

Prolonged poor posture, any lack of mobility, or poor recovery from injury, initiates adaptive shortening of tissues around a joint which then leads to dysfunction. The shortened tissues give pain whenever they are stretched into what would have been normal range.

Think of your finger again. If it is never straightened from a slightly bent position up to the limit of its range in any exercise or activity for years, in time the structures in the front of the joint will shorten and stiffen, eventually preventing movement beyond the small range of daily use. This may not seem to matter for your finger function but it is very important for other joints such as knees and hips where large ranges are necessary for efficient and comfortable use – and for backs. We need supple, mobile spines for healthy living.

Soft tissue shortening occurs, for example, in the 'dowager hump' posture, a kyphotic deformity usually related to degenerative changes in the cervico-thoracic junction (Greive, 1988), and in the poking-chin stance (**4.5**). In the latter case abnormal lengthening and shortening takes place in quite a complicated pattern in the cervical spine. Similar problems can be present in any part of a stiff spine or, in fact, in any joint of the body that is not used in its full range.

Dysfunction manifests in the form of stiffness and intermittent pain at the end of movement range. The joints are vulnerable, they lack full function and are thus susceptible to any other injury.

4.5

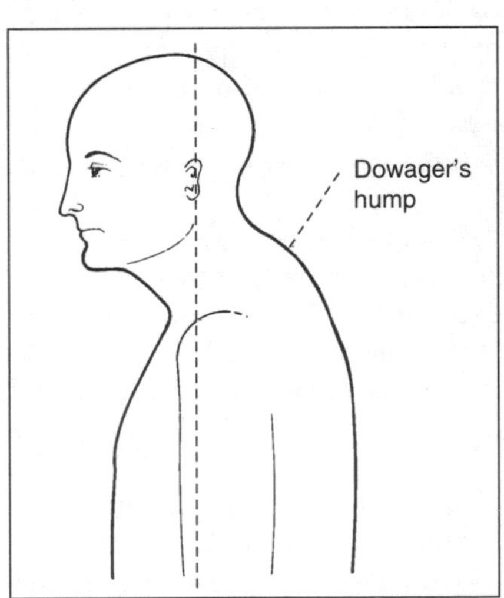

4.5. 'Dowager hump' and poking chin

Trauma

The term 'sprain' in relation to the vertebral column is open to dispute. Research to date finds no evidence of the pathology of sprain occurring in the back (Bogduk and Twomey, 1991). It is, however, a useful term to illustrate a clinical picture which depicts a series of signs and symptoms which cannot be accurately ascribed to any particular tissue of the back but which closely resembles the signs and symptoms evoked by a peripheral joint sprain, for example a sprained ankle, something experienced by most people (Bogduk, 1992).

Sprain of a peripheral joint occurs as a result of sudden trauma, often of a twisting nature but always involving a stressed or unbalanced range of movement. It can result from an apparently insignificant gesture or a larger action, but there is immediate pain. The degree of damage may vary from a 'tweak' of the ligamentous and capsular tissue to a major tear of the fibres, sometimes involving the cartilage, but invariably there is trauma to surrounding tissue with resulting swelling, inflammation and pain.

Comparable symptoms are evoked in the vertebral column by sudden movement, stretching, lifting, twisting or from the trauma of accident. There is acute pain, intermittent or constant, with or without limb referral; muscle spasm may be present, causing a temporary scoliosis. Swelling is not often visible in the back as the soft tissues are hidden by the musculature, but it can be palpated around the lumbo-sacral area at times. Heat is certainly palpable.

The most common 'sprain' of the 20th century is whiplash, the violent backward-forward thrust of the head in a car accident. It involves not only the cervical spine but also the upper thoracic and can embroil the whole vertical column, compromising ligamentous, capsular, cartilaginous, discogenic, muscular, vascular and nervous tissues even to implicating the sympathetic nervous chain (Butler, 1991).

Whiplash-type injuries can occur in sport, for example in diving, in the sudden explosive movement of a tennis serve, or in the same flexion-extension action of bowling in cricket. Constantly loading the spine in extension can affect the point of impact of the extended Z joints, giving rise to a sclerosis and thickening of the compact bone of the lamina often observed in young adult spines (Twomey *et al.*, 1988).

Sprain-type injuries can involve multiple joints, as in a whiplash or lifting accident, or just one joint if 'tweaked' while performing a minor movement. They can also be the harbinger of discogenic problems. Diagnosis can only be deduced by the specific signs and symptoms of the pain together with careful examination.

Joint derangement

Joint derangement can include anything causing a malfunction within a joint – it could be a bulging intervertebral disc or a 'locked' Z joint. A discogenic problem can elicit pain ranging from slight to severe low back pain, with pain, paraesthesia and/or anaesthesia in the leg, with varying degrees of neurological involvement. The character of the pain is in itself an aid to diagnosis (see Chapter 7, p. 96–97). Mobilisation and back care are successfully used in treatment, depending on the degree of derangement.

A 'locked back' can occur with minor bending movements. The back becomes fixed in flexion, with the sufferer unable to move out of it. It is thought to be caused possibly by a cartilage entrapment in one of the Z joints, or possibly nuclear material lodged in the outer annulus. It is often a painful condition but manipulative techniques are usually successful in relieving it (Taylor and Twomey, 1987).

Inflammation

Inflammation can occur in the joints of the spine as a result of:

- Any injury.
- An infection. This can be from something as simple as a viral infection, such as 'flu, or from a septicaemic condition, or from certain fevers such as typhoid.
- Disease, for example, rheumatoid arthritis, tuberculosis or osteomyelitis.

Inflamed joints are hot, swollen and red, though redness, like swelling, is not often visible in the spine.

Treatment for all these clinical presentations is based on the signs and symptoms of the patient's tissue disturbances, with the aim of reducing pain, from whatever cause, and restoring function.

In the mobile human being the bones provide the skeletal structure, the joints allow mobility whilst the ligaments and capsules control undue range. The whole is a truly mechanical system of levers and hinges. The next chapter deals with the pulleys which initiate and perform movement: the body musculature.

REFERENCES

Adams, M.A. and Hutton, W.C. (1982). Prolapsed intervertebral disc: a hyperflexion injury, *Spine*, **7**(3), 184–191.

Adams, M.A. and Hutton, W.C. (1985). Gradual disc prolapse, *Spine* **10**(6), 524–531.

Bogduk, N. (1986). Review paper, the anatomy and pathophysiology of whiplash, *Clin. Biomech.*, **1**(2) 92–101.

Bogduk, N. (1992). The sources of low back pain, *The Lumbar Spine and Back Pain* (Jayson, M.I.V., ed.), 4th ed, Churchill Livingstone.

Bogduk, N. and Twomey, L.T. (1991). *Clinical Anatomy of the Lumbar Spine*, 2nd ed, Churchill Livingstone.

Butler, D. (1991). *Mobilisation of the Nervous System*, Churchill Livingstone.

Butler, R.C. and Kerr, M. (1992). Rheumatoid arthritis and juvenile chronic arthritis, *Cash's Textbook of Orthopaedics and Rheumatology for Physiotherapists*, Mosby-Year Book Europe.

Crock, H.V. (1986). Internal disc disruption: a challenge to disc prolapse fifty years on, *Spine* **11**(6), 650–653.

Dixey, J.J. and Kerr, M. (1992). The spondyloarthropathies, *Cash's Textbook of Orthopaedics and Rheumatology for Physiotherapists* (Tidswell, M.E. ed.), Mosby Year Book Europe.

Galasko, G.S.B. (1992). Back pain in children, *The Lumbar Spine and Back Pain* (Jayson, M.I.V, ed.) 4th ed, Churchill Livingstone.

Grennan, D.M. and Jayson, M.I.V. (1984). Rheumatoid arthritis, *Textbook of Pain* (Wall, P. and Melzack, R. eds.), Churchill Livingstone.

Greive, G. (1988). Common vertebral joint problems, 2nd ed, Churchill Livingston (page 379).

Harkness, J.A.L., Higgs, E.R. Dieppe, P.A. (1984). Osteoarthritis, *Textbook of Pain* (Wall, P. and Melzack, R. eds.), Churchill Livingstone.

Hickey, D.S. and Hukins, D.W.L. (1980). Relation between the structure of the annulus fibrosus and the function and failure of the intervertebral disc, *Spine,* **5**(2), 106–117.

Lipson, S.J. (1988). Metaplastic proliferative cartilage as an alternative concept to herniated intervertebral disc, *Spine*, Vol. 13, No. 9.

Markolf, K.L. and Morris, J.M. (1974). The structural components of the intervertebral disc. *J. Bone Joint Surg.*, **56A**(4), 675–687.

McKenzie, R. (1981). *The Lumbar Spine, Mechanical Diagnosis and Therapy*, Spinal Publications.

Mixter, W.J. and Barr, J.S. (1934). Rupture of the intervertebral disc with involvement of the spinal canal, *N Engl J Med*, 211: 210-215.

Mooney, M.D. and Robertson, J. (1976). The facet syndrome, *Clin. Orthop.*, **115**, 149–156.

Mourad, L.A. (1991). *Orthopedic Disorders*, Mosby–Year Book.

Nathan, H. and Israel, J. (1962). Osteophytes of the vertebral column, *J Bone Joint Surg.*, **44A**(2), 243–264.

Panjabi, M.M. and White, A.A. (1980). Basic biomechanics of the spine, *Neurosurgery*, 7(1),76–93.

Taylor, J.R. and Twomey, L.T. (1987). The lumbar spine from infancy to old age, *Physical Therapy of the Low Back* (Twomey, L.T. and Taylor, J.R. eds.), Churchill Livingstone, USA.

Taylor, J.R. and Twomey, L.T. (1986). Age changes in the lumbar zygapophyseal joints, *Spine,* **11**(7), 739–745.

Twomey, L. (1991)(personal communication). *Lumbar Intervertebral Discs.*

Twomey, L.T. and Taylor, J.R. (1987). Age changes in the lumbar vertebrae and the intervertebral discs, *Clin. Orthop.*, **221**(224), 97–103.

Twomey, L.T. and Taylor, J.A. (1991).Age-related changes in the lumbar spine and spinal rehabilitation, *Critical Reviews in Physical and Rehabilitation Medicine,* **2**(3), 153–169, Printed by CRC Press Inc.

Twomey, L.T., Taylor, J.R. and Oliver, M.J. (1988). Sustained flexion loading, rapid extension loading of the lumbar spine, and the physical therapy of related injuries. *Physiotherapy Practice,* 129–137, Longman Group UK Ltd.

Vernon-Roberts, B. (1992). Age-related and degenerative pathology of intervertebral discs and apophyseal joints. *The Lumbar Spine and Back Pain* (Jayson, M.I.V., ed.), 4th ed, Churchill Livingstone.

Ward D.J. and Tidswell, M.E. (updated by Dixey, J.J. and Kerr, M.) (1992). Osteoarthritis, *Cash's Textbook of Orthopaedics and Rheumatology for Physiotherapists,* Mosby-Year Book Europe.

Yasuma, T. , Ohno, R. and Yamauchi, Y. (1988). False-negative lumbar discograms, *Journal of Bone and Joint Surgery*, Vol. 70-A, No. 9.

Yasuma, T., Koh, S., Okamura, T. and Yamauchi, Y. (1990). Histological changes in ageing lumbar intervertebral discs, *Journal of Bone and Joint Surgery*, Vol. 72-A, No. 2.

5. The muscles of the back

Muscular shape and outline

A muscle is a fleshy, contractile, elastic pulley which facilitates body movement. The contours of the body outline are shaped by the substance of muscles, especially those of the buttocks and limbs. Body builders make an art of developing each superficial muscle to sculptured perfection, and adopt certain poses which isolate and display particular muscle bulk as it contracts.

Muscles vary in shape. They can be spindle-shaped, thinner at both ends with one end tapering down to a tough sinewy tendon, as in the calf muscles, or they can be flattish sheets like some muscles of the back. Muscles also range in size from the long, tough visible muscles of the thigh to the short, intricate, invisible muscles deep in the neck. Muscles are attached to bone at crucial places above a joint and are inserted into other bone on the far side of the joint. The mechanism can be further complicated by the muscle passing over more than one joint, having a different effect on each.

The structure of muscle tissue

There are three kinds of muscle tissue – skeletal, smooth and cardiac. Skeletal or striped muscles function under voluntary control and are concerned with body movement, they contract and relax on command; the smooth or unstriped muscle tissues of the internal organs work without conscious control; cardiac muscle is a mixture of the two – involuntary but striped (Ganong, 1991; Mourad, 1991). Only skeletal muscle will be discussed in this book.

Skeletal muscle is made up of individual muscle fibres, each of which is a long cylindrical cell of **sarcoplasm** surrounded by a membrane, the **sarcolemma**. The fibres are separated from each other by delicate connective tissue known as the **endomysium** and are bound together into bundles or **fasciculi** by a dense covering, the **perimysium**. The groups of fasciculi which form the whole muscle are enclosed by a fibrous covering, the **epimysium**. The three connective tissues provide pathways for nerves and blood vessels supplying the muscle cells (Ganong, 1991; Mourad, 1991; Palastanga, 1991).

Muscular contraction

Stimulation

Muscle cells can be excited chemically, electrically and mechanically to produce an action potential that is transmitted along their cell membrane (Ganong, 1991). The stimulus occurs at a motor end plate (see Chapter 6, p. 79) and the action potential is transmitted along the muscle fibre, initiating a contractile response (Ganong, 1991; Mourad, 1991)).

A single action potential causes a brief muscle contraction known as a muscle **twitch**. Repeated stimulation before relaxation has occurred creates a **summation of contraction**. Rapid repeated stimuli elicit a **tetanic contraction**, causing complete tetanus when there is no relaxation at all (Ganong, 1991).

In the intact human or animal, healthy skeletal muscle contracts only in response to stimulation of its motor nerve. Destruction of its nerve supply causes muscle atrophy; it can also lead to excitability of the muscle and fine irregular, invisible **fibrillations** (contractions of individual fibres) appear. These disappear when the nerve regenerates (Ganong, 1991).

The motor unit

The smallest amount of muscle that can contract in response to stimulation is not one single muscle fibre but all the fibres supplied by a motor neurone. Each single motor neurone and the fibres it supplies are a **motor unit.**

The number of fibres in each unit vary, for example, muscles with fine graded movement, such as the hand, have 3–6 muscles fibres per unit; large muscles can have as many as 165. There are slow and fast motor units depending upon the speed of their contractions. Slow motor units are innervated by small, slowly-conducting motor nerves, and fast units by rapidly-conducting large motor nerves. The small slow units are recruited first in most movements as they are resistant to fatigue and are the most frequently used units. The fast units which are more easily fatigued are generally recruited with more forceful activities.

The differences between types of motor units are not inherent but are determined by the central nervous system. There is little response in skeletal muscles at rest; with minimal activity a few motor units discharge, and with increasing effort more and more are brought into play. This process is called **recruitment of units** (Ganong, 1991).

The strength of any contraction is determined by the number of motor units in action and the number of times per second that each unit is stimulated. Muscle cells either respond entirely to a stimulus or not at all. A stimulus strong enough to bring about a contraction is called a **liminal** stimulus; a less intense stimulus is **subliminal** (Mourad, 1991). When a liminal stimulus is received, all fibres of a motor unit contract.

Types of muscle contraction

A muscle contraction can be isotonic or isometric:

- **an isotonic contraction** is one in which the muscle shortens and fattens, pulling its two ends closer together, eliciting movement of the joint or joints over which it passes.
- **an isometric contraction** is one in which tension is developed but no change of length takes place, usually because of contracting against resistance.

Muscles contracting isotonically have the ability to work in opposite directions, working **concentrically** as they shorten, **eccentrically** as they 'pay out'

Rest your hand and forearm on the table, palm down, and look at your fingers and forearm. Lift and lower one finger and as you do so watch the tendon moving on the back of the hand. Follow the movement up your forearm and you will see the muscle rippling just below the elbow; play around with all your fingers and the movements become quite lively. The fleshy part below the elbow is the belly of these muscles, the finger extensors, and as they contract, shortening and fattening, they *pull* the fingers back, working concentrically. To return the fingers to the table the muscles *pay-out*, working eccentrically lowering the fingers in a controlled manner.

If you now turn your hand over and bend your fingers you will be using the muscles on the front of your forearm, the flexors of the fingers.

Each joint has controlling muscle groups, the **prime movers**, which move it in one direction and an opposing group, the **antagonists**, which move it the opposite way. Muscles which control movement while others are working are **synergists**. In normal movements the synergists act as stabilisers, keeping a limb steady while other muscles work dynamically to perform the action. This occurs a great deal in joints of multiple movement like the shoulder and in postural control of the back while movement occurs in the limbs.

The **quadriceps muscles** and **hamstring muscles** are the two groups which work around the knee (**5.1**) – the quadriceps straighten the knee on contraction and the hamstrings bend it. The **back extensor muscles** and the **abdominal muscles** are the two controlling groups of the trunk.

Muscle contraction resulting in a change of length of the muscle is **isotonic**; a static muscle contraction in which tension is developed but no movement takes place is **isometric.**

5.1

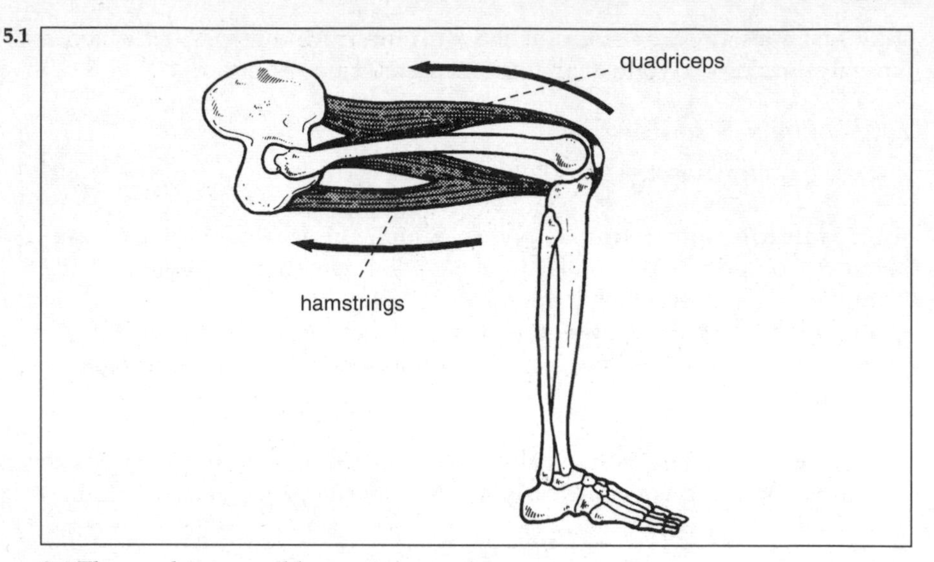

5.1 The quadriceps and hamstring muscles

However, muscle balance or imbalance is more complex than the simple interplay between muscle groups; new concepts incorporate principles affecting the relationship between muscle length and muscle tension, motor control and recruitment, joint biomechanics and neural control (Comerford, 1993).

The muscles of the trunk

Although the detailed anatomical knowledge of back musculature is necessary for surgeons or therapists when treating patients, it is not relevant in the context of back care. This chapter will look mainly at the functional elements of the two groups of muscles concerned with the back, the **back extensor muscles** and the **abdominal muscles**.

Stripped of its musculature, the vertebral column is wholly unstable. The muscles provide support for the spine, control movements of the whole vertebral column and stabilise vertebral posture during work or movement of the limbs (Troup, 1979; Panjabi *et al.*, 1989).

The back muscles

The muscles of the back are in three layers, separated by and attached to the **thoracolumbar fascia** (see below). The deepest layer consists of short muscles attached from one vertebra to another repetitively up the spine; the second layer consists of longer muscles travelling over several vertebrae; and in the most superficial layer are the longest and largest muscles, attached to the pelvis in the lower back, the thoracic and cervical spine and the scapula (shoulder blade) at the top. These are the muscles which are clearly visible on certain trunk and strong arm movements (**5.2**).

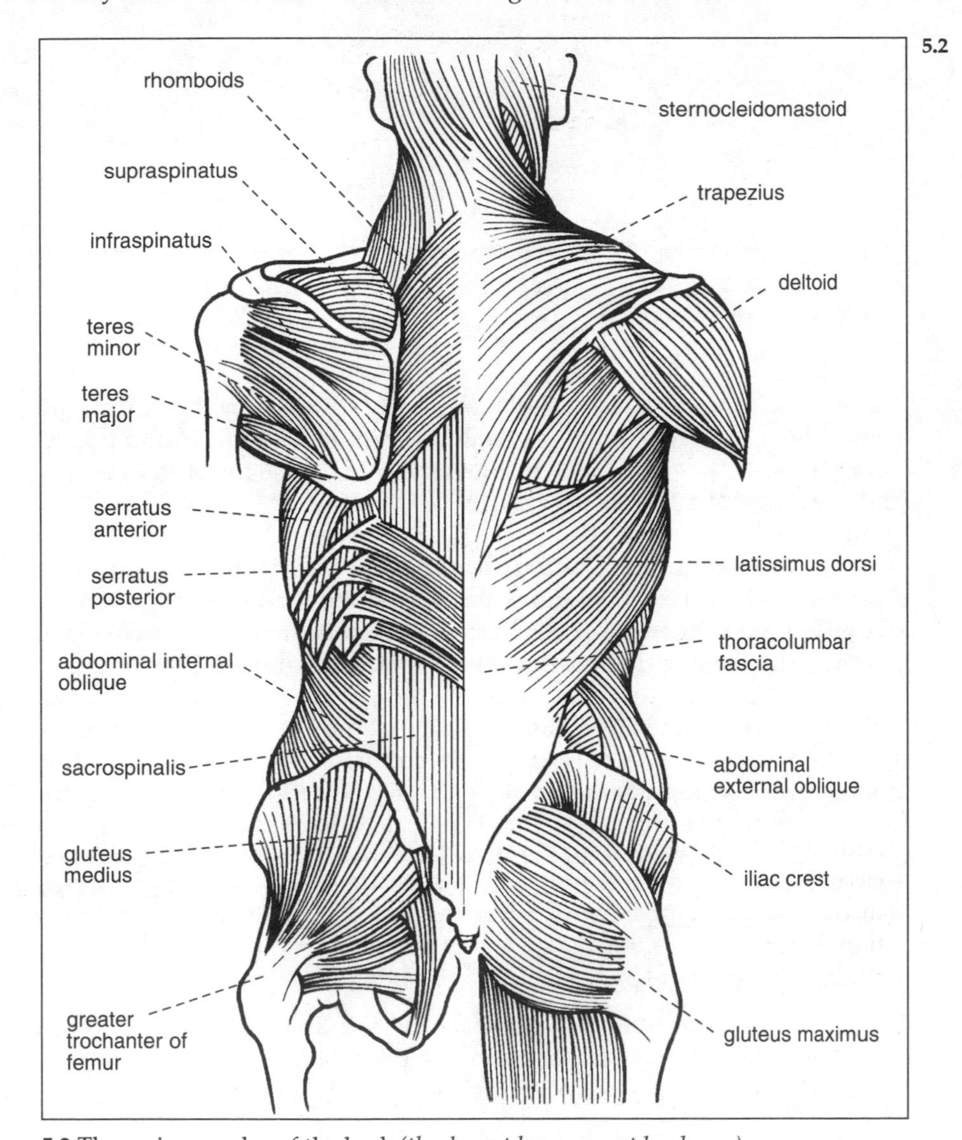

5.2 The main muscles of the back *(the deepest layer cannot be shown)*

The vertebral attachments of these muscles are on the posterior elements of the vertebrae. As they contract they pull on the vertebrae, initiating movement in the desired direction and exerting considerable stress upon the pedicles. The diversity of size and attachment of these muscles enables the body to perform minor movements of intricate adjustment as well as major changes of trunk position.

Lying prone (face down) the back muscles work to extend the back, raising the shoulders from the floor (**5.3**).

5.3

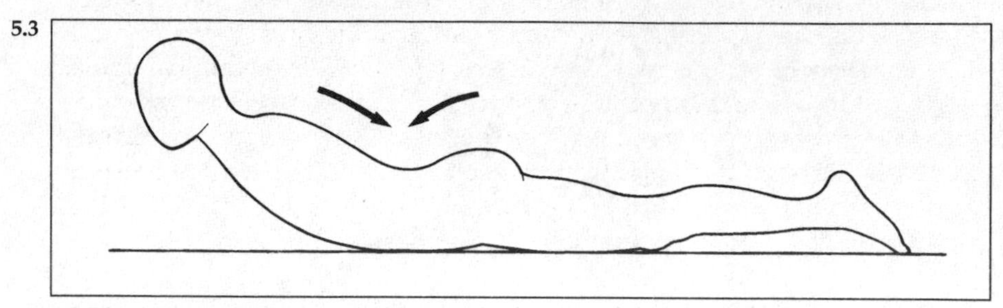

5.3 The back extensor muscles

In the erect posture they work constantly to keep the back upright against the tendency of gravity to pull it down. In forward bending they work eccentrically, paying-out to allow the trunk to be lowered in a controlled way against the pull of gravity.

At a certain point in forward flexion, activity of the back muscles ceases and the vertebral column is braced by the locking of the Z joints and by tension in their posterior ligaments (McIntosh and Bogduk, 1987) together with tension of the thoracolumbar fascia (Sullivan, 1989).

As the movement changes into an active extension from the bent position, the muscles work concentrically to raise the back. Because the muscles are working parallel to the spine in the action of extension, the force of contraction exerts a longitudinal compression on the spine (Bogduk and Twomey, 1991). *This is an important aspect to consider in rehabilitation of the back after injury, as excessive compression in exercises might need to be avoided.*

The muscles of the abdomen

There are five abdominal muscles each performing different functions (Johnston, 1945); but, unless training enables isolation of their action, they work together and perform in unison as a supportive unit.

Rectus abdominis is the flat central muscle attached to the pubic crest and ligaments of the pubis below, and to the ribs and sternum above; its main action is flexion of the spine and rigidity of the abdominal wall.

Pyramidalis is a small muscle below rectus abdominis attached to the pubis and the **linea alba** (the central line of fascia running down the centre of the abdomen, through the umbilicus); it assists flexion of the lower abdomen by tensing the linea alba.

The **internal** and **external oblique** and **transversus abdominis** are attached at the back to the thoracolumbar fascia, below to the iliac crest and the **inguinal ligament** (which runs from the anterior superior iliac spine to the pubis), above to the ribs and centrally to the abdominal fascia and the linea alba. The two oblique muscles working together flex the lumbar spine, assist in respiration and support the abdominal contents; working independently they rotate the trunk on the pelvis. Transversus abdominis compresses the abdomen and stabilises the linea alba. These three muscles are used in dynamic abdominal bracing or 'back bracing', described in Chapter 18, p. 194, and in abdominal hollowing on p. 201.

There are also four major muscles of the posterior abdominal wall, at the back of the abdomen but in front of the vertebrae; **quadratus lumborum**, **psoas major** and **minor**, and **iliacus**. The psoas muscles are attached to the lumbar vertebral bodies and discs at one end and the femur at the other (Johnston, 1945). Contraction of the psoas muscles flexes (bends) the hip, pulling the knee towards the chest; in episodes of back pain this is often, not surprisingly, a difficult and pain-provoking movement.

Lying supine (flat on the back), contraction of the abdominal muscles brings the ribs nearer to the symphysis pubis, and brings the chest towards the groin in a straight movement of flexion or a sit-up (**5.4**)

5.4

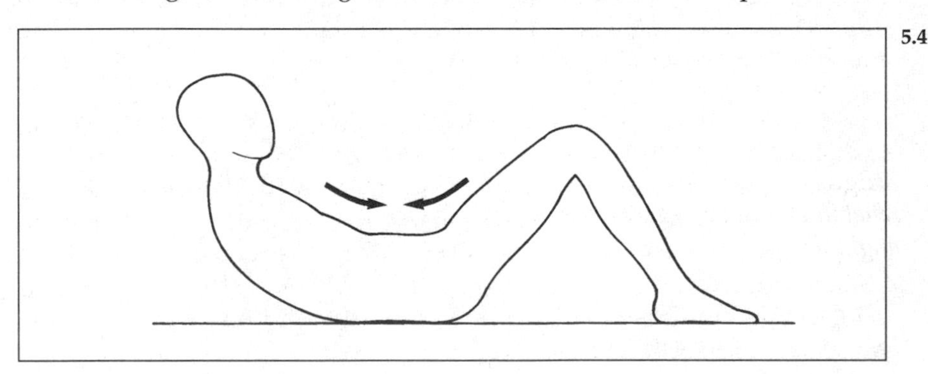

5.4 The abdominal muscles

Thoracolumbar fascia

The thoracolumbar fascia consists of three layers of fascia effectively separating the three muscular layers of the lumbar spine. The layers of fascia are attached to the spinous processes, the transverse processes, the intertransverse ligaments (between the transverse processes) and the ligamentous attachments of the muscles; the fascia reinforces the posterior ligamentous system through the orientation of its fibres (Kisner and Colby, 1990).

Passive tension in the posterior layer occurs with lumbar flexion, the increased tension supporting the lower lumbar vertebrae by stabilising them against the forces of flexion (Bogduk and Twomey, 1991). Activity of the muscles attached to or surrounded by the fascia increases the tension of the fascia which in turn increases support of the lumbar spine (Kisner and Colby, 1990). Recent studies show that the thoracolumbar fascia provides a major support mechanism in the act of lifting (Sullivan, 1989).

The control of movement and posture

Gravity

Movement is never as simple or as clear-cut as in **5.1**, **5.3** and **5.4**. Gravity influences every action we make and dictates the role played by muscle groups throughout the body. As we move in different directions the muscles of the thorax are working eccentrically or concentrically to hold or correct any position.

In the upright position gravity tends to pull us down, to bend the knees, bend the hips and collapse the shoulders towards the pelvis. The leg muscles have to keep constant watch to maintain straight legs without forcing the knees back into a locked position; the hip muscles must maintain straight hips without pressing them into a forward thrust; and the back extensor muscles have to juggle with the abdominal muscles to support the spine while the neck muscles steady the head on top. The muscles involved are the 'anti-gravity' muscles.

Think what happens to our heads when we grow sleepy while sitting upright. The head falls and flops about in all directions. The muscles of the neck respond by trying to haul it back to the neutral upright position. In the waking state this is a continuous, unnoticed process. Certain muscles, by making constant tiny corrections in all directions, hold the head still with static work while other muscles turn it in the direction we consciously require. This unceasing interplay between muscle groups is the muscular mechanism of posture.

Muscular recruitment

Inputs from the brain converging on motor units serve three functions:

- They bring about voluntary action.
- They adjust body posture to provide a stable background for movement.
- They coordinate the action of the various muscles to make movements smooth and precise (Ganong, 1991).

Anatomically, each muscle functions predominantly as either a stabiliser or a mobiliser, although certain activities may demand a change of role.

Physiologically, muscle fibres can be recruited tonically or phasically. **Tonic fibre recruitment** characteristics are slow-twitch fibres, slow to contract, slow to fatigue, with a strong sensory feedback. These are used as stabilisers of movement and anti-gravity control. **Phasic fibre recruitment** characteristics are fast-twitch fibres, fast to contract, fatiguing quickly, able to perform rapid, repetitive movements. These are used for mobilising actions and rapid ballistic movements (Comerford, 1993). Ideally, stabilising muscles should be used primarily for tonic fibre recruitment and mobilising muscles mainly for phasic recruitment.

Postural problems

Adaptive responses in muscle (changes in function and structure) take place:

- As a result of recruitment reversal: when stabilising muscles are recruited phasically and mobilising muscles are recruited tonically.
- As a result of poor posture or a sedentary lifestyle.

Joint dysfunction is the inevitable result.

Recruitment reversal: in activities of the limbs, the muscles of the trunk are primarily postural stabilisers, controlling the hips and pelvis while activity takes place in the arms and legs (Richardson et al 1992). If for any reason, for example joint stiffness or poor working postural habits, there is loss of movement in the hips and shoulders, movement of the back is substituted. Examples of this occur when:

- Undue pelvic movement is substituted for hip flexion and extension in walking.
- Shoulder girdle movement is substituted for pure arm movement in certain repetitive occupations, such as production line work.

Poor posture: in poor posture stabilising muscles 'give' and no longer control ideal vertebral alignment; the upper trunk muscles and the oblique abdominals are those which tend to weaken more easily (Richardson, 1992). The result is an alteration of the correct postural curves and an adaptive change in opposing muscle groups. This occurs, for example, with 'round shoulders' where the muscles of the thoracic spine and shoulder girdle slacken and lengthen while those of the pectoral region (the front of the chest) shorten and tighten; or with the increased lordosis when the abdominal muscles slacken and the back extensions are tight.

When overload, in the form of work or sport, is added to muscle imbalance, the spine becomes vulnerable to injury (Sahrmann, 1987).

Re-education of muscle strength

The strength of a muscle is directly related to its length (Comerford, 1993). Alteration in the length, by posturally allowing it to elongate or shorten adaptively, will relatively either weaken or strengthen the muscle.

Similarly, over-development of one group of muscle by excessive exercise can lead to shortening and tightening of those muscles with lengthening and weakening of their opposing group (ibid 1993). Lengthened muscles must be shortened with exercise and shortened muscles must be stretched (ibid).

Most people manage to preserve the strength and ability of the lumbar back extensor muscles, often purposefully exercising them, but the abdominal muscles suffer a sad decline early in life, a deterioration often prompted merely by sloppy standing postures when they are no longer used as stabilisers and all tone is lost. Abdominal muscles also weaken when there is poor recovery from pregnancy, poor recovery after abdominal operation, or in obesity. Over-eating or heavy beer drinking drags the abdomen forwards mechanically, as does pregnancy, allowing the weight of the stomach content to promote sagging of the muscles, mechanically handicapping their contraction.

Unlike the back extensors, the abdominal muscles are not used automatically in daily activity. All sorts of trick movements are employed to avoid exerting them. For example, when did you last make yourself sit up from lying in bed by using your stomach muscles and not by pushing yourself up with your arms? After slouching in an armchair, when did you last make yourself sit forwards without pulling on the chair arms with your hands? When did you last try to pull and hold your abdomen in while standing?

The last action – hollowing the abdomen with a sustained, gentle contraction is one of the most re-educative exercises to restore muscle balance in posture (see Chapter 18, p. 201).

Muscles can be strengthened by:

- Slow, sustained, maintained contraction as in postural correction, which shortens and strengthens weak long muscles and stretches shortened ones.
- Repetitive strengthening exercises.

Postural corrections are covered in detail in Chapter 11. These corrections should be held and maintained repetitively throughout the day. Specific muscular control exercises, for example abdominal hollowing, should also be practised. Repetitive strengthening exercises, when necessary, should be performed for any weak muscle group, ensuring that when balance is achieved all groups are equally activated.

It has been proven that the stresses and strains of muscular activity actually strengthen bone and that a lack of exercise leads to a decrease in strength and health generally, leaving the spine vulnerable (Twomey and

Taylor, 1991). Weightlifters not only protect their backs from injury by postural care, but their backs actually protect themselves. The vertebrae adapt to the rigorous training by becoming more robust as the muscular strength increases (Bogduk and Twomey, 1991). There is also strong evidence to suggest that although there appears to be a decline in strength during the process of ageing, this is by no means inevitable (Twomey and Taylor, 1991).

Keeping all muscles strong should be an important regime in the prevention of back trouble. All that are required are a few brief exercises every day, ensuring a balanced approach to all groups, combined with meticulous postural correction and a resolve to grab every opportunity to use the body fully.

Disorders of muscles

Muscles are intended for hard, tough work, but they can be damaged and, when not functioning accurately, can be the cause of dysfunction.

Muscular imbalance

Changes in muscle function play an important role in the contributory factors of many painful conditions of the back and constitute an integral part of postural defects in general (Comerford, 1993). Muscular balance leads to precise movement and musculo-skeletal health; muscle imbalance leads to movement dysfunction and tissue trauma (ibid).

Strains, sprains, tears and ruptures

Muscle strain results from over work, either by working for too long or by sustaining too heavy a load. **Muscle sprain**, tears or rupture result from sudden movement, either because the muscle was unprepared for the movement or because the demand was too great for its ability. Neck muscles can be sprained in whiplash injuries, as can back muscles when lifting is wrongly performed or when lifting an over-heavy load. Muscular tears and ruptures are rare in back injuries except as a result of severe trauma, but they are quite common in sports injuries involving the limbs.

Spasm or cramp

There are many causes of muscle spasm and cramp. They are both involuntary contractions, without conscious control. **Muscle spasm** implies a reflex contraction of muscle surrounding an inflamed or injured structure (Mills *et al.*, 1989). It is frequently encountered in back conditions, commonly referred to as 'protective spasm'. It occurs as a sustained, involuntary contraction, usually of the muscles of one side of the back which deviate the spine out of alignment. By preventing all movement the body seems to believe it can avoid pain – hence the term 'protective' –

but the action is often counter-productive. The muscles may be painful when this occurs, but they are not necessarily part of the injury. Muscle spasm also occurs in certain neurological conditions.

Muscle cramp is also an involuntary contraction. There are several causes, some chemical (from a decrease in body salts and potassium), some ischaemic (a blockage of blood supply), some neurological. Cramp occurs most frequently in the calf muscles and is a hazard for athletes (Mills *et al.*, 1989).

Weakness of muscle

Muscular weakness can exhibit in two different ways: an inability to achieve the required strength, which could be related to muscular denervation, or an easy, rapid fatigue which implies impaired blood supply (Mills *et al.*, 1989).

Denervation can be the result of any neurological condition; in relation to the back, denervation occurs when a nerve root has been damaged sufficiently to reduce conductivity. The muscles supplied by the affected nerve weaken and waste in size. If nerve regeneration is possible, the muscle will recover but full restoration can take some time.

Muscular inflammation

Direct trauma to muscular tissue can result in bruising and a local inflammatory reaction. Muscular inflammation can also occur in certain systemic conditions such as polymyalgia rheumatica (Mills *et al.*, 1989).

Muscular pain

Two kinds of muscle pain occur in association with exercise (Mills *et al.*, 1989):

- Pain occurring during exercise which stops as soon as movement ceases. This is due to ischaemia or loss of blood supply to the muscle. Intermittent claudication and angina pectoris are two clinical presentations of this condition but it can occur, and does occur, in any muscle occluded of its blood supply; for example, in a hand after carrying a heavy case or after maintaining any repetitive fast exercise.
- Pain felt hours after exercise which may persist for days. This is associated with especially strong eccentric muscle activity which can damage muscle if performed too hard or for too long (Mills *et al.*, 1989).

After recovery from any injury muscles must be gradually stretched and strengthened to restore full function.

So, by concentric, eccentric or static work, muscles enable the skeleton to perform extraordinary manoeuvres in a precise and intricate manner, from picking up a speck of dust to balancing the entire body in the most complicated gymnastic dance. All this would be quite impossible without the control of the nervous system centred in the brain.

REFERENCES

Bogduk, N. and Twomey, L.T. (1991). *Clinical Anatomy of the Lumbar Spine*, 2nd ed, Churchill Livingstone.

Comerford, M. (1993) (personal communication).

Ganong, W.F. (1991). *Review of Medical Physiology*, 15th ed., Appleton and Lange.

Johnston, T.B. (ed.)(1945). *Gray's Anatomy*, Longmans, Green and Co., England.

Kisner, C. and Colby, L.A. (1990). *Therapeutic Exercise. Foundations and Techniques*, 2nd ed, F. A. Davis, Philadelphia.

Mourad, L.A. (1991). *Orthopedic Disorders*, Mosby Year Book.

McIntosh, J. and Bogduk, N. (1987). The anatomy and function of the lumbar back muscles and their fascia, *Physical Therapy of the Low Back* (Twomey, L.A. and Taylor, J.R. eds.), Churchill Livingstone, USA.

Mills, K.R., Newham, D.J. and Edwards, R.H.T. (1989). Muscle pain, *Textbook of Pain* (Wall, P.D. and Melzack, R. eds.), 2nd ed., Churchill Livingstone.

Palastanga, N., Field, D. and Soames, R. (1991). *Anatomy and Human Movement*, Heinemann Medical Books.

Panjabi, M., Abumi, K., Duranceau, J. and Oxland,T. (1989). Spinal stability and intersegmental muscle forces: a bio–mechanical model, *Spine*, **14**, 194–200.

Richardson, C., Jull, G., Toppenberg, R. and Comerford, M. (1992). Techniques for active lumbar stabilisation for spinal protection: a pilot study, *Australian Physiotherapy*, **38**(2).

Sullivan, M.S. (1989). Back support mechanisms during manual lifting, *Physical Therapy*, **69**(1), 36–45.

Sahrmann, S.A. (1987). Muscle imbalance in the orthopaedic and neurological patient. *Proceedings of the 10th International Congress of the World Confederation for Physical Therapy*, Sydney, 836–841.

Troup, J.D.G. (1979). Biomechanics of the vertebral column, *Physiotherapy*, **65**(8), 238–244.

Twomey, L.T. and Taylor, J.R. (1991). Age related changes of the lumbar spine and spinal rehabilitation, *Physical Rehabilitation and Medicine*, **2**(3), 153–169, CRC Press Inc.

6. *The nerve supply of the back*

General mechanism

The human nervous system is the most highly developed and complicated in the whole animal kingdom. Its structure and function are intricately bound together (Bowsher, 1988). The system really needs to be considered as one, as it is a continuous tract throughout the whole body. It is a continuum in three ways:

- The connective tissues are continuous.
- The neurones are connected electrically, so that an impulse generated at the foot is received in the brain.
- The system is continuous chemically, the same neurotransmitters exist peripherally as centrally and there is a flow of cytoplasm inside axons (Butler, 1991).

However, for the sake of description it is divided into three parts: the central nervous system, the peripheral nervous system and the autonomic nervous system.

The central nervous system

The central nervous system (CNS) consists of the **brain** and the **spinal cord**. Detailed knowledge of their structure and function is not essential for the understanding of back pain, so only an outline is given here.

The **brain** contained within the skull is protected by the cranial bones and by three membranes: the **dura mater** on the outside, the **arachnoid mater** in the middle and the **pia mater** on the inside. The brain, like a specialised computer, absorbs all the data fed into it from the various senses, stores the information, analyses new experience in the light of previous learning and then instructs the body about any necessary action to be taken. It contains grey matter – cell bodies which receive, store and transform messages, and white matter – the nerve fibres which transmit the messages.

The **spinal cord**, contained within the spinal canal of the vertebral column, is the central transmitting station. It becomes continuous with the brain at the **foramen magnum**, the exit from the skull. The spinal cord consists of a central core of grey matter around which the white matter is arranged, all surrounded and protected by the same membranes as the brain. The dura mater of the spinal cord is a tough fibrous tube which is continuous with the cranial dura and descends down to the level of the sacrum. It is the toughest of the three sheaths and is separated from the wall of the canal by fatty pads and a plexus of veins. Between the arachnoid mater and the pia mater is the **subarachnoid space** containing **cerebrospinal fluid** (Johnston, 1945) (**6.1**).

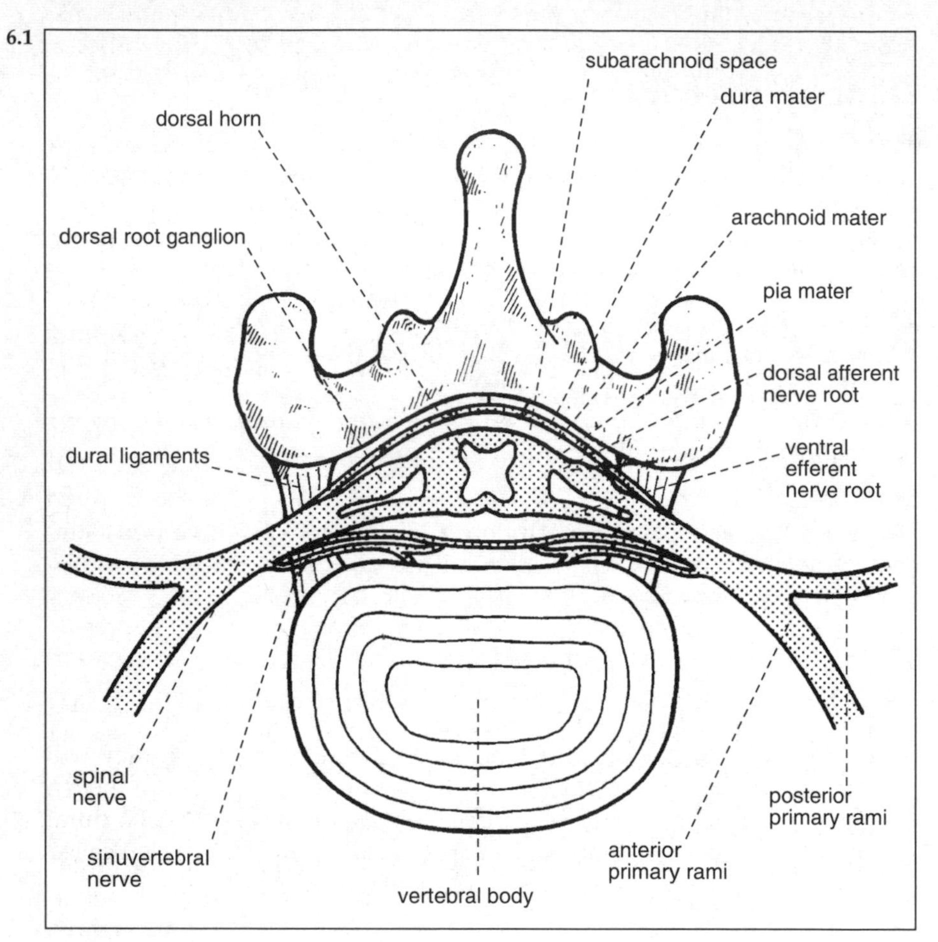

6.1 The contents of the spinal canal

The spinal cord is suspended within the canal and tethered to the bony structures by dural ligaments (Butler, 1991). In the upright or extended posture it hangs in a relaxed wavy line; on extreme flexion the cord elongates in the canal, moving forwards as it does so (Breig and Marions, 1962; Breig and El-Nadi, 1964; Troup, 1986). From extreme spinal extension to complete flexion the spinal canal lengthens from 5–9cm (Butler, 1991). The changes in length and volume of the canal between flexion and extension, lateral flexion to each side and rotation lead to major changes in the resting tension of the cord (Breig, 1978). The ability of the cord to elongate within the canal on movement is highly relevant to the subject of spinal and neural mobility and to the subject of **adverse neural tension** which will be discussed later.

From the foramen magnum the spinal cord travels down through the canal for about 45cm to the level of the first or second lumbar vertebra, where it ends, tapering to a cone shape forming the **conus medullaris**. From this point a delicate non-nervous filament, the **filum terminale**, descends to anchor the cord at the first coccygeal segment (Johnston, 1945).

Pairs of **nerve roots** emerge from either side of the cord at appropriate levels of the cord's grey and white matter: an anterior and a posterior root. The anterior or ventral nerve root carries efferent or motor nerve fibres, which convey messages of activity to the structures of the body; the posterior or dorsal nerve root carries mainly afferent or sensory fibres conveying messages of sensation from the body to the CNS. Each root is covered with its own sleeve of pia mater which is continuous with the pia mater of the spinal cord (Bogduk and Twomey, 1991).

The cervical nerve roots leave the cord level with their exit through the intervertebral foramen (IVF). However, as the spinal cord is shorter than the spinal canal, the roots' emergence further down the cord no longer coincides exactly with their final exit; by the time the cord ends at the second lumbar vertebra, the lumbar and sacral nerve roots have already emerged from the cord and the mass of nerve roots, known as the **cauda equina** or horse's tail, descend in a cluster towards the sacrum, *still enclosed in the dural sac* (Johnston, 1945).

Just above the level of the intervertebral foramen from which they will exit the pair of roots pierce through the dura mater and, taking with them a continuation of the dura mater and arachnoid mater in the form of a dural sleeve, they pass down towards the relevant IVF in a soft tissue canal called the **radicular** or **intervertebral canal** (Bogduk and Twomey, 1991).

At the IVF the dorsal and ventral nerve roots unite to form a **spinal nerve**, but just before doing so the dorsal root develops a bulge, the **dorsal root ganglion**, which contains the cell bodies of the sensory nerve fibres (see **6.1**). The dura mater becomes the **epineurium** or outer covering of the spinal nerve after they unite (Hewitt, 1970).

The spinal nerve is usually very short, only as long as the width of the IVF, and contains motor and sensory nerve fibres and fibres from the autonomic nervous system. The spinal nerve immediately divides into two branches, the smaller posterior or dorsal rami and the larger anterior or ventral rami, which become the peripheral nerves of the body. Immediately after its formation the ventral ramus gives off the

sinuvertebral nerve, which re-enters the intervertebral foramen to become the nerve supplying all the vital structures within the spinal canal (see **6.1**). Thus the dura mater, the dural sleeve of the nerve roots, the sheaths of the spinal nerves, the posterior longitudinal ligament, the annulus fibrosis, the blood vessels of the spinal canal and the periosteum (the outer covering of bone) of the vertebral bodies all become pain-sensitive structures within the spinal canal (Butler, 1991).

The peripheral nervous system

The peripheral nervous system consists of 12 cranial nerves and 31 pairs of peripheral nerves. The **cranial nerves** leave the brain inside the skull and travel directly to the eyes, ears, mouth, face and parts of the head. The **peripheral nerves** are a continuation of the spinal nerves. Some travel directly to their ultimate destinations while others link up with other nerves to form plexuses (groups of nerves) which divide and subdivide until they reach the extremities of the fingers and toes.

The nerve supply to the areas of the body is quite logical: the nerves from the upper cervical spine supply the head and neck; those of the lower cervical and upper thoracic spine join to form the **brachial plexus** which runs down the arms; the thoracic nerves supply the ribs, abdomen and the trunk; the lumbar and sacral nerves join to form the **lumbar** and **sacral plexuses** which supply the lower trunk and legs.

Some nerves are surprisingly large to start with; the sciatic nerve which runs all the way down the back of the leg is as thick as a finger but by the time it splits into the numerous nerves necessary to cover all the cutaneous areas of the skin, these final nerves are mere threads.

In their sensory role nerves serve certain specific areas of the body; these areas can vary slightly from person to person but, on the whole, for example, if skin sensation is deficient over the front of the thigh, there is likely to be a problem with the second or third lumbar nerve. In their motor capacity nerves innervate muscle tissue and evoke voluntary response, supplying specific muscles, so, for example, a weakness of the quadriceps muscles could help to corroborate a nerve root problem at L3.

The autonomic nervous system

The autonomic nervous system is made up of the **sympathetic** and **parasympathetic** nervous systems. They are antagonists in their effect, the sympathetic excites and the parasympathetic inhibits (Walton, 1989). The nerve fibres are distributed to the internal organs such as the various glands, viscera, blood vessels and involuntary muscles of the body organs. (Palastanga *et al.*, 1991).

The fibres of the **sympathetic nervous system** travel down through the spinal cord, exiting with the spinal nerve between the first thoracic and second lumbar vertebrae, to form a sympathetic chain on either side of the vertebral column from the base of the skull to the coccyx (Butler, 1991; Ganong, 1991; Palastanga *et al.*, 1991).

It has been found that the sympathetic chain can be affected by flexion/extension movements of the vertebral column and can be damaged by violent trauma as in whiplash injuries (Butler, 1991).

The **parasympathetic nervous system** includes cranial and sacral outflow. The cranial parasympathetic nerves supply the head, heart, lungs and upper part of the body and the sacral nerves the lower organs and tissues. Although the parasympathetic nerves travel in the mixed peripheral nerves they are not part of the sympathetic chain (Johnston, 1945; Ganong, 1991; Palastanga *et al.*, 1991).

The autonomic nervous system is greatly influenced by our emotions and *vice versa*. Excitement causes the heart to beat faster; anger starts the adrenalin flowing, increasing energy for action; fear dries up the mouth. We are often quite unaware of the subtle changes taking place. Butler (1992) is now putting forward the hypothesis that trauma to the sympathetic nervous system might possibly in turn create great emotional disturbance by chemical means.

Nerve structure, nerve endings and impulse transmission

Nerve structure

The basic unit of the nervous system is the **neurone**. All neurones have three characteristic components: a **cell body**, **dendrites** and an **axon** (the nerve fibre).

The **cell body** contains the nucleus and apparatus necessary to sustain the metabolic activities of the cell (Palastanga *et al.*, 1991). Cells are located in the grey matter of the brain and the spinal cord and in certain ganglia like the ganglia of the dorsal nerve root. The motor nerve fibres originate from the cell bodies of the ventral horn of the spinal cord and terminate at neuromuscular junctions; the sensory nerve fibres originate from the cell bodies of the dorsal root ganglia and terminate at sensory receptors or as free nerve endings in the tissues (Sunderland, 1978; Lundborg, 1988).

Dendrites are short branching processes which radiate in various directions from the cell body. They are responsible for receiving information from other nearby cells and transmitting it to the cell body (Bond, 1984; Ganong, 1991; Palastanga *et al.*, 1991).

The **axon** is a longitudinal, tubular extension of the cell membrane composed of a core of cell cytoplasm or axoplasm surrounded by a multi-layered sheath (Sunderland, 1978). The axon or nerve fibre is the basic structure which carries the nerve impulses and also transports vital chemicals in the axoplasm along its entire length (Melzack and Wall, 1991; Butler, 1991). The axoplasmic flow travels through the axonal transport system of the nerve fibre in both directions and three main flows have been identified (Lundborg, 1988; Butler, 1991). The maintenance of this flow is vital, not only for the health of the nerve which depends upon its' relationship with the cell body, but also for the health of the tissues it supplies, the 'target tissues' (Sunderland, 1978; Butler, 1991).

An adult has tens of thousands of axons to supply the foot alone and the tubular axons run all the way to the foot from the spinal cord without interruption – a distance of 1 metre (Melzack and Wall, 1991).

Each **peripheral nerve** contains bundles of nerve fibres, sensory, motor and autonomic; each bundle or fascicle contains a huge number of fibres. The fibres are protected by three layers of connective tissue: the endoneurium around the axon, the perineurium around each fascicle and the epineurium surrounding the whole nerve with its fascicular bundles (**6.2**). The sheaths act as a protective cover for the sensitive conductive axons in the centre and contain blood vessels for the supply of nutrients.

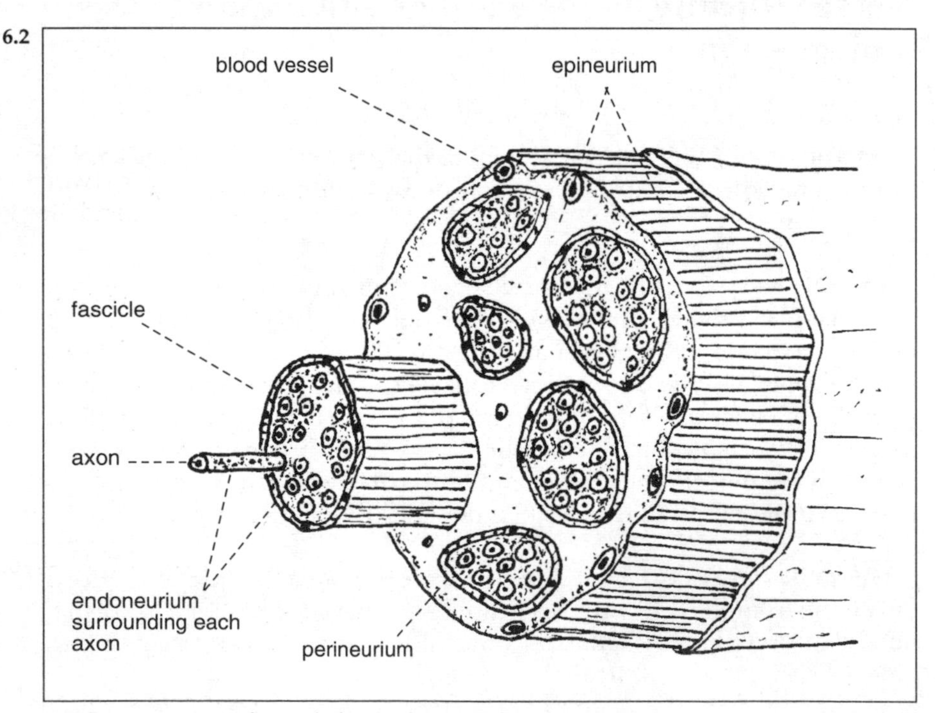

6.2 Cross-section of a multifascicular peripheral nerve

Nerve endings

The nerve endings are in the actual tissues of the body, in the skin, the muscles, the ligaments, joint capsules, organs of the abdomen (liver, kidneys, etc.), in the outer coverings of the blood vessels, and in the neural tissue sheaths (Butler, 1991). However, neither the vertebral end plate nor the inner portion of the disc is supplied with nerves, so two major load-bearing structures of the back can be damaged without eliciting pain. All other tissues of the motion segment receive a nerve supply and are thereby able to communicate their responses to the brain.

Motor nerve endings deliver stimuli to muscle fibres at the neuromuscular junction complex known as the **motor end plate**. (Palastanga *et al.*, 1991).

Sensory nerve endings, or receptors, in the tissues are complex and are of many different kinds. They respond to touch, pressure and thermal changes; **mechanoreceptors** in the joints respond to change of position, supplying information about joint movement; muscle tissue contains free nerve endings (which register pain) and two kinds of receptors: **Golgi** tendon organs (which monitor the extent of muscle contraction) and **muscle spindles** (which monitor changes in muscle length) (Palastanga *et al.*, 1991); while **nociceptors** in all tissues react to noxious stimuli of any kind, so registering pain.

Impulse transmission

Nerve conduction. Impulses are transmitted from one nerve cell to another at junctions or **synapses**. Transmission at most synaptic junctions is chemical, the impulse from the axon causing secretion of chemical neurotransmitters. Synapses typically occur between the axon of one neurone and the dendrite of another, but they can be between axons and cell bodies, axons and axons or even dendrites and dendrites (Palastanga *et al.*, 1991).

Sensory axons are of different sizes and they transport impulses at different velocities. They are traditionally divided into three groups: fast A-beta or large myelinated fibres, slightly slower A-delta or small myelinated fibres, and slow C unmyelinated fibres; about 60% of all afferents are in the C group (Melzack and Wall, 1991). Myelin is a sheath present in some nerves which increases the speed at which impulses can be conducted. These fibres all respond to different degrees of stimulation, briefly: A-beta for free light pressure, vibration and joint position, A-delta for pin-prick and fast pain, some pressure, temperature and chemical irritation, and C fibres which respond most readily to noxious stimuli and carry slow pain.

Put your finger behind your back and waggle it around. You cannot see what you are doing but you know what is happening. How? You know because the receptors in the tissues, the skin and joints are informing you of every movement and change of position. You can even discern exactly what you are touching behind your back, providing it is something your brain can recognise from past experience. If you touch something hurtful, you react immediately by withdrawing your hand and perhaps registering pain or displeasure.

The reflex arc is a short-cut system which the body uses in emergencies. If we touch something hot, the sensation is transmitted along the sensory nerve in the usual way and enters the grey matter of the spinal cord in the dorsal horn, but instead of the message being passed on to the brain it is shot across into the ventral horn where motor impulses initiate immediate action. Awareness of the message only occurs after action has been taken. Although the reflex action is not totally conscious it is still within conscious control.

The blood supply of the nervous system

The nervous system consumes 20% of available oxygen in the circulating blood yet makes up only 2% of body mass (Bowsher, 1988; Butler, 1991; Ganong, 1991). Nerve cells are especially sensitive to alteration in blood flow so an uninterrupted blood supply is imperative for the metabolic demands of normal neural function (Butler, 1991). The vertebral column has a rich supply of blood vessels supplied by the lumber arteries and veins, giving off fine branches to all tissues (Dommisse and Grobler, 1976; Crock and Yoshizawa, 1976). They pass in and out of the IVF which becomes a gateway for all structures entering or leaving the spinal canal. So the spinal cord, nerve roots and the peripheral nerves are well supplied with nutrients both to their outer coverings and to the inside of the nerve tissue.

Disorders of the neural tissue within the spinal canal

Any disorder of the nervous system must involve at least one of the two relevant neural tissues: impulse conductive tissue and protective, supportive tissue (Butler, 1991).

This book only considers those disorders of the neural tissue within the spinal canal and the nerves related to spinal problems, not diseases or disorders of the central nervous system.

The most common disorders associated with vertebral problems are the mechanical and physiological consequences of stretch, friction and compression (Butler, 1991). The two major factors in the resulting pathology are mechanical and vascular dysfunction, and, as nerves are dependent upon an uninterrupted supply of blood for normal function, the vascular factors seem to be of greater importance (Sunderland, 1978; Lundborg, 1988).

The central structures in the spinal canal need space and anything which jeopardises this can lead to nerve root problems or disturbance of the structures within the spinal canal. This space must be adequate during rest and during movement (Troup, 1986).

Neural tissue impingement

Nerve roots and neural tissue can be impinged upon by any offending object such as oedema (swelling) of surrounding tissue, a bulging intervertebral disc, an osteophyte or other bony impingement of the vertebral canal or intervertebral foramen, or restriction by scar tissue (Troup, 1986). Any abnormality which stretches or increases the resting tension of nerve roots can lead to ischaemia (blockage of blood supply), pain and diminished conductivity. The impingement can lead to irritation or compression.

Nerve irritation

Nerve irritation can result from chemical irritation such as the inflammatory response from a nuclear extrusion, or from the mechanical trauma of repeated injury, for example impingement of an osteophyte or a bulging intervertebral disc. Epineural oedema can result from quite mild compression or friction (Rydevik *et al.*, 1984). Irritation of nerve tissue results in pain and sometimes in subjective feelings of paraesthesia and anaesthesia without actual loss of sensation.

If the irritation and inflammation persists, the intraneural tissues may be affected which is potentially damaging to the nerve fibre itself and can result in loss of conductivity (Lundborg, 1988).

Nerve compression

Nerve compression can be acute or chronic:

- Acute compression can result from a severe, abrupt, transient impingement (Sunderland, 1978).
- Chronic compression or **entrapment neuropathy** occurs when a nerve is slowly or even intermittently compressed until the nerve fibres are destroyed and the nerve tissue is converted into fibrous tissue (ibid).

Compression of neural tissue results in paraesthesia followed by loss of conductivity, resulting in loss of sensation and weakness. Compression of the dorsal root ganglion leads to pain, but pain is only elicited in the nerve roots when there is also damage to the nerve tissue (Bogduk and Twomey, 1991). Ischaemia is usually a component of nerve compression which can lead to irreversible damage (Breig and Marions, 1962; Sunderland, 1978).

The most common cause of compression is **spinal stenosis**. There are three canals in the spinal vertebrae: the spinal canal, the intervertebral canal and the canal through the IVF. Narrowing or stenosis can occur in any or all of these canals. It may be local, segmental or generalised. It may be caused by bone or soft tissue or any space-occupying lesion and the narrowing may involve the bony canal alone or the dural sac or both (Arnoldi *et al.*, 1976; Porter, 1992). Apart from alteration of the shape and size of the canal, compression can result from: buckling of the ligamentum flavum, osteophytes on the vertebral bodies or Z joints, or disc bulges and herniations. Depending on the level of the stenosis, the narrowing can cause pressure on the spinal cord or the cauda equina, compression of the nerve roots or entrapment of blood vessels. (Kirkaldy-Willis, and McIvor, 1976). There can be loss of conductivity in the nerve supply to a limb, with symptoms of neurogenic claudication – intermittent paraesthesia and anaesthesia, often without pain (Porter, 1986). If the symptoms are caused by narrowing of the spinal canal, they are often relieved by bending into flexion; the converse frequently applies if the symptoms are caused by intermittent claudication of vascular origin, when flexion tends to increase the symptoms.

Adverse neural tension

During the movements of the body through flexion and extension the spinal cord is elongated in the spinal canal producing tension and movement in the nerve roots (Breig and Marions, 1962). We are becoming more aware of the quantity of movement which takes place in the neural environment during everyday living, not only of the cord within the spinal canal and the roots within the IVF but also of the peripheral nerves within their mechanical interface tunnels throughout the body during flexion and extension movements of the limbs, the mechanical interface being any structure adjacent to the nervous system (Butler, 1991). The peripheral nerve trunks are not fixed to the surrounding tissue but, with movement, they slide longitudinally within their interface (Lundborg, 1988).

David Butler, in *Mobilisation of the Nervous System* (1991) defines adverse neural tension as:

> *'abnormal physiological and mechanical responses produced from nervous system structures when their normal range of movement and stretch capabilities are tested'.*

These abnormal responses are seen clinically as limitation of movement within the nervous system which can be demonstrated by tests which stretch the nervous tissue – the straight-leg-raise, the prone-knee-bend, the slump, the cervical-neck-flexion and the upper-limb-tension tests investigate various aspects of the movement of neural tissue within the body and within the spinal canal. The tests give some guide to the degree of neural involvement in the area.

However, these tests have superceded their original diagnostic purpose and are now fully integrated into therapeutic techniques whenever pathology affects the normal biomechanics of the nervous system. Physiotherapy would include treatment of the interface tissues and careful mobilisation of the nerve limitation (Butler and Gifford, 1989).

Adverse neural tension is a commonly-encountered element in all spinal disorders which have related limb symptoms. It is also too frequently ignored as a cause of the continuation of spinal or limb pain after the acute phase is over.

The important roles of the nervous system are to keep the body functioning and to tell us what is happening; to convey messages of daily activity, of precise movement, of pleasure, of discomfort. In the latter role it is the lifeguard at the lookout post, watching what is happening out of sight 'behind our backs', and ready to blow the whistle of warning – pain.

REFERENCES

Arnoldi, C.C., Brodsky, A.E., Cauchoix, J., *et al.*, (1976). Lumbar spinal stenosis and nerve root entrapment syndromes, *Clin. Orthop,*. **115**, 4–5.
Bogduk, N. and Twomey, L.T. (1991). *Clinical Anatomy of the Lumbar Spine,* 2nd ed., Churchill Livingstone.
Bond, M.R. (1984). *Pain. Its nature, Analysis and Treatment,* 2nd ed., Churchill Livingstone.
Bowsher, D. (1988). *Introduction to the Anatomy and Physiology of the Nervous System,* 5th ed., Blackwell Scientific Publications.
Breig, A. (1978). Adverse mechanical tension in the central nervous system, *Almquist Wiksell International,* Stockholm.
Breig, A. and Marions, O. (1962). Biomechanics of the lumbosacral nerve roots, 72. 633038 *Acta Radiologica,* Vol. 1, Diagnosis, 1141–1160.
Breig, A. and El-Nadi, A.F. (1964). *Biomechanics of the Cervical Spinal Cord.* From the Centre of Neurosurgery, UAR Armed Forces Hospital, Cairo, Egypt, 16 August, 602–623.
Butler, D. (1991). *Mobilisation of the Nervous System,* Churchill Livingstone, Singapore.
Butler, D. (1992) (personal communication). *Lecture on Mobilisation of the Nervous System.*
Butler, D. and Gifford, L. (1989). The concept of adverse mechanical tension in the nervous system, *Physiotherapy,* November, **1**(75), no.11.
Crock, H.V. and Yoshizawa, H. (1976). The blood supply of the lumbar vertebral column, *Clin. Orthop.,* **115**, 6–21.
Dommisse, G.F. and Grobler, L. (1976). Arteries and veins of the lumbar nerve roots and cauda equina, *Clin. Orthop.,* 115.
Ganong, W.F. (1991). Review of Medical Physiology, 15th ed., Appletone and Lange.
Johnston, T.B. (ed.) (1945). *Gray's Anatomy,* Longmans, Green & Co, England.
Hewitt, W. (1970). The intervertebral foramen, Moira Packenham-Walsh Foundation Lecture, *Physiotherapy,* **August**, 332–335.
Kirkaldy-Willis, W.H. and McIvor, G.W.D. (1976)(co guest eds.) Lumbar spinal stenosis, *Clin. Orthop.,* **115**, 2–3.

Lundborg, G. (1988). *Nerve Injury and Repair*, Churchill Livingstone.
Melzack, R. and Wall, P. (1991). *The Challenge of Pain*, Penguin Books.
Palastanga, N, Field, D. and Soames, R. (1991). *Anatomy and Human Movement, Structure and Function*, Heinemann Medical Books.
Porter, R.W. (1986). *Management of Back Pain*, Churchill Livingstone.
Porter, R.W. (1992). Spinal stenosis of the central and root canal, *The Lumbar Spine and Back Pain*, Jayson, M.I.V. (ed.), 4th Ed., Churchill Livingstone.
Rydevik, B., Brown, M.D., Lundborg, G. (1984). Pathoanatomy and pathophysiology of nerve root compression, *Spine*, **9**, 7–15.
Sunderland, S. (1978). *Nerve and Nerve Injuries*, 2nd ed., Churchill Livingstone.
Troup, J.D.G. (1986). Biomechanics of the lumbar spinal canal, *Clinical Biomechanics*, **1**(1), 31–43.
Walton, Lord (1989). *Essentials of Neurology*, 6th ed., Churchill Livingstone.

7. *Pain*

The mystery of pain

Pain is the most complicated area of human experience. Understanding it is a challenge to medicine, to the sufferer and to society (Melzack and Wall, 1991). Although in recent years new concepts regarding all aspects of the complex mechanisms of pain, a certain mystery still remains.

Perhaps the enigma stems from our wide use of the word to describe all suffering, from the mild sensation of a pinprick to the agony of bereavement to the relentless pain of an incurable disease. Hidden within this spectrum there are associations with punishment, with martyrdom, with the intimation that stoicism leads to inner strength, that 'it must get worse before it gets better': that pain is inflicted on us and we are the victims of its aggression.

The origin of this attitude lies in the word itself. 'Pain' is derived from the Greek *poine* (a tax) and the Latin *poena* (a punishment or penalty) (Fabrega and Tyma, 1976); the latter had both physical and mental implications in classical Latin. Thus the mind–body links in the word are present from its very earliest appearance in language and, from the beginning, our word 'pain' had an association with wrongdoing (ibid).

The description of pain is rooted in historical and cultural factors. Religious and moral beliefs, age and gender all affect the individual's interpretation and response to pain. Culture includes the distinctive features of a person's entire lifestyle, and as such shapes psychological experience and social behaviour (ibid).

Another perplexing factor in our understanding of pain lies in the complicated relationship between injury and the degree of pain it elicits. Certain conditions defy straightforward physiological explanations of pain:

- **Congenital analgesia** is a condition in which there is an inability to feel pain, yet the nervous system is intact.
- **Episodic analgesia** is a condition in which there is a lack of feeling at the time of injury (Beecher, 1959; Melzack and Wall, 1991).

Conversely, there are cases of severe pain in the absence of injury or long after injury has healed (Melzack and Wall, 1991). Thus injury may occur without pain and pain without injury.

Definitions of pain

Pain is a symptom which humanity has tried to understand in terms of religion, philosophy and medicine from time immemorial (Fordham, 1992). The International Association for the Study of Pain (1979) defines pain as *'an unpleasant sensory and emotional experience associated with actual or potential tissue damage or described in terms of such damage'*.

Pain is not a primary sensation – as are vision, hearing, touch, smell and thermal sensitivity – but an emotional disturbance resulting from the development of mechanical and/or chemical changes in body tissue of such nature and magnitude that they activate afferent systems that are normally quiescent (Wyke, 1976). No matter how bizarre the clinical presentation, pain is always indicative of some degree of dysfunction (ibid).

'Pain is whatever the experiencing person says it is, and it exists wherever he says it does' (McCaffery, 1972). The fundamental point of reference for the nurse's approach to pain is the patient's subjective experience of pain.

The psychology of pain

Psychological evidence refutes the one-to one-relationship between stimulus and sensation. The same injury can have different effects on different people and on the same person at different times (Melzack and Wall, 1991).

The purpose of pain

There is much controversy about the purpose pain serves:

- According to Sternbach (1989), pain enables the organism to sense impending tissue damage and so avoid harm and prolong survival. Evidence supporting this comes from studies of people with congenital insensitivity to pain who have short life spans as a result.
- On the other hand Leriche (1939) denounces the concept of pain as a useful warning signal: *'Physicians too readily claim that pain is a reaction of defence, a fortunate warning, which put us on our guard against the risks of disease...Defence reaction? Fortunate warning? But as a matter of fact, the majority of diseases, even the most serious, attack us without warning...'*

It is true that irregularities of pathology can occur without pain. Cancer (referred to by Leriche) elicits no pain unless the tumour starts to impinge upon other pain sensitive tissues. However, this fails to alter the fact that pain, when it does occur, usually signals tissue disorder.

The nature of pain

The role of pain as a messenger changes depending on its duration. Never a harbinger of good tidings pain is, in its briefest appearance, a helpful warning; in its longest display it becomes a self-perpetuating reminder of an insoluble situation, making pain appear to *be* the aggressor instead of the *outcome* of some form of assault.

Pain can be divided into three types, according to its duration: transient pain, acute pain and chronic pain (Melzack and Wall, 1991).

Transient pain is passing. In most injuries it is unimportant. A finger pinched in a door will elicit a sharp stab of pain for a short while but little or no damage has been done and there is no anxiety. The pain is quickly forgotten (Melzack and Wall, 1991).

Acute pain is transient pain that does not go away. The characteristics of acute pain are the combination of tissue damage, pain and anxiety (Melzack and Wall, 1991). But acute pain has a well-defined course with a characteristic time span with pain disappearing after the course of healing (Weisenberg, 1989). The timescale of injury and healing is a precise one (see Chapter 8, p. 101).

Chronic pain. The greatest challenges to pain relief are concerned with chronic pain (Fordham, 1992). Defining chronic pain presents one of the greatest difficulties; perhaps each definition adds to the picture as a whole. Carpenito (1983) defines chronic pain as persistent or intermittent pain that last for more than six months (Fordham, 1992). Melzack and Wall (1991) define it as pain that begins as acute pain but which lasts after healing has taken place; it often becomes a pain syndrome and a medical problem in its own right.

The persistence of chronic pain may be associated with low-level abnormal sensory inputs that produce self-sustaining neural activity; these inputs are memory-like mechanisms related to pain, known as pattern generating mechanisms (Weisenberg, 1989). Normally these mechanisms are inhibited by a central controlling system; when neural damage occurs, for example in an amputation or a peripheral nerve lesion, the central inhibitory mechanisms can be diminished (see modulation of pain, below), thus allowing sustained activity to occur even as a result of non-noxious input as, for example, in phantom limb pain.

Whatever the reason for its existence, while acute pain may promote survival (by its warning mechanisms), chronic pain is usually destructive physically, psychologically and socially (Sternbach, 1989). The uncertainty of the origin of pain seems to be one of the most disturbing factors for the sufferer; in contrast, people with known and diagnosed incurable diseases seem not to follow the same pattern of depression, disability and invalidism as other chronic pain sufferers, unless the pain finally becomes intolerable (ibid).

The difficulty for both the patient and the clinician is to be certain that healing has taken place. The failure of self-healing mechanisms together with failed efforts at self-management and conventional medical care can leave a patient severely debilitated. Emotional and behavioural disturbances can result (Craig, 1984).

Psychogenic pain

When psychological factors appear to play a predominant role in a person's pain, the pain may be labelled as 'psychogenic'. The person is presumed to be in pain because he needs or wants it (Melzack and Wall, 1991). Hysteria and hypochondriasis are grouped in this class. McCaffery (1972) says that repression of conflicts is a major factor in hysterical pain, and that hypochondriacal pain is thought to be based on failed passed experiences. However, Melzack and Wall (1991) believe that chronic pain is usually the cause rather than the result of neurotic symptoms.

The conscious perception of pain

Emotional influences: The conscious perception of pain is greatly influenced by the prevailing emotional state. Diversion of attention reduces pain, albeit temporarily. Anxiety and preoccupation with pain magnifies the intensity. These observations are related to the strange phenomenon that allows the toleration of greater degrees of pain in moments of crisis. In an emergency, in war or sport for example, pain can be blocked off for hours to enable the person to continue with the essential job at the time. Soldiers have been known to have legs blown off with apparently little regard to their plight until the next day – although they still reacted to the pain of an injection at the field hospital (Beecher, 1959). Beecher believed this to be possible because of the soldiers' euphoria at being alive, but Melzack and Wall (1991) feel the phenomenon is not yet fully explained.

Verbal reports of personal pain frequently focus on emotional discomfort, expressing feelings of displeasure and anguish, with the use of evocative terms such as 'exhausting, frightening and sickening' (Craig, 1984).

The most common concomitants of painful discomfort are anxiety, fear and depression, though other emotions may extend through to anger, aggression, subservience, sexual arousal and even laughter (ibid). Anxious people are particularly vulnerable to pain but fear, anxiety and depression are also capable of amplifying pain (Bond, 1984). Anxiety and depression may also provoke an autonomic nervous system visceral and skeletal activity which may exacerbate pain (Craig, 1984).

French (1989) and McCaffery (1972) report that patients find it helpful to be given information about their pain, and that understanding can help to allay fear and anxiety. Egbert *et al.*, (1964) found that patients given information about post-operative pain required significantly less analgesia after surgery, and made a quicker recovery than those who had not been advised. However, care must be taken not to give wrong or worrying information because knowledge alone may increase anxiety due to the expectation of pain it can create (French, 1989).

Involving patients in self-appraisal and control over their emotional states, while helping them to choose the most appropriate way of coping with pain, is part of the nursing approach to patients in pain (Fordham, 1992). It should be the attitude of all health care workers, with a change of accent depending on the particular field of medicine concerned.

Memory patterns: Emotionally traumatic life experiences and past experiences with pain become memory patterns which influence all other stimuli (McCaffery, 1972). McCaffery quotes Pavlov (1927) who found that alarm and defence reactions could be initiated by any stimulus that had been previously associated with injuries, dangerous threatening situations or frustrations. In this way sufferers of child abuse may have an unspoken hurt which remains part of every painful experience (Butler, 1992).

Cultural, religious and social influences on pain perception: McCaffery (1972) quotes Zborowski (1969): *'The fear of pain is said to rank only second to the fear of death.'* However, in some cultures and religious sects pain is regarded as morally elevating, or, when self-inflicted, as a means of expiating feelings of guilt attached to some supposed transgression (Wyke, 1976). There are many initiation rites which involve painful rituals where the participants feel no pain at all (Melzack and Wall, 1991). Stoicism is an attitude to pain which is reflected in certain cultural groups more than others and in certain family attitudes; age and gender often determine the acceptability of certain deviations from the norm within a group, with girls often allowed greater freedom to express pain than boys (McCaffery, 1972).

Describing and measuring pain

Describing and quantifying pain can be confusing.The perception of pain and pain complaint are not necessarily synonymous; it is possible to be in considerable pain and yet hide it from others, or to complain a great deal even though the pain is minimal (French, 1989).

Describing pain: Melzack and Wall (1991) point out the difficulties in scientifically measuring the language of pain. However, in a clinical situation, despite all the personality variations that may be present, it is astonishing how consistently people of one language and culture use the same adjectives to describe their pain, building up a meaningful picture. Within an English-speaking group 'severe', 'stabbing', 'dull ache', 'burning', 'throbbing', 'crawling', 'shooting' are some of the regular definitions. Some people manage to find uniquely evocative descriptions, but ones which are immediately recognisable to the listener.

The quality of pain as expressed by the patient may well be an important guide to diagnosis (Melzack and Wall, 1991); this is especially relevant in musculoskeletal conditions.

However, as the language, culture and religion of individuals greatly affects their attitude towards illness, and the way in which they tolerate pain, the description of that pain may only be fully appreciated by people of the same group (Fabrega, 1976).

Measuring pain: 'pain thresholds' have been used to explain people's different reactions when quantifying pain. There is now evidence that the majority of people, regardless of background, have a uniform **pain sensation threshold**, that is the least intensity level at which a sensation is first felt. However, the **pain tolerance threshold**, the greatest intensity that a subject can bear, is a greatly variable factor being related to upbringing, past experience, expectations of bravery and to cultural background (Hardy, 1952; Zborowski, 1952; Sternbach and Tursky, 1965; Bowsher, 1988a).

The physiology of pain

A noxious stimulus received by the nociceptors in the tissues is converted into energy which is carried along different-sized nerve fibres at varying speeds to the dorsal horn of the spinal cord and thence transmitted to the brain. However, pain only becomes pain when it is perceived as such by the brain, and at any level of transmission pain can be modulated.

Modulation of pain

Modulation means that information from a receptor can be changed, enhanced, diminished or even suppressed, either at the periphery or in the central nervous system (Bowsher, 1988a).

Enkephalins, endorphins and dynorphins are all endogenous pain inhibitors which are manufactured in the grey matter of the brain and are present in the dorsal horn (Fields and Bausbaum, 1984; Porter, 1986; Melzack and Wall, 1991). Thus afferent stimulus is modified by descending chemicals from the CNS.

Drugs can also be used to affect pain at a wide range of sites along nociceptive pathways, acting against the pathological processes producing pain at the periphery to modulation of the response at cerebral level (Baxter, 1988).

Local anaesthetics act by stabilising the membranes of nerve c blocking the generation of impulses so that the nerve remains in its resting state (Melzack and Wall, 1991).

In 1965 Melzack and Wall proposed a new theory – **the Gate control theory** – which has revolutionised the concept of pain. Prior to this there were two theories of pain physiology:

- **Specificity theory** is a sensory theory which proposes that pain is a sensory phenomenon in its own right with special receptors, special routes of transmission through the central nervous system, and special centres for registration, appreciation and interpretation in the brain (Hayward, 1981; Bond, 1984).
- **Pattern theory** stems from a group of theories formed as a reaction against the specificity theory. An intensity theory emerged which says that specific receptors for pain do not exist and that pain arises as a result of stimulation by any means, so long as the intensity of that stimulation passes a certain threshold (Bond, 1984).

The Gate control theory incorporates elements of both these theories but also takes into account the role played by emotion in the experience of pain and attitude towards it. The grey matter of the dorsal horn of the spinal cord is the collecting centre for sensory input to the brain. Sensitive messages arriving there are either shot straight across into the ventral horn for a reflex action or they are transmitted up to the brain for recognition and action. But at this point the messages can be modified by two sources before they evoke pain perception:

- Descending inhibitory messages from the brain.
- Other more powerful stimulation from large sensory nerves (Melzack, 1982).

The analogy of the 'gate' arises from the picture evoked by the small-fibred nerves carrying messages of pain which, if uninterrupted, 'open' the gate in the dorsal horn for the transmission up to the brain where pain is 'recognised'. The messages can be modified,and the gate thus 'closed', by descending inhibitory messages from the brain (including previously learned responses) or by messages from the mechanoreceptors in muscles and joints sending messages along the large sensory nerves. Sensory input is therefore subjected to the modulating influence of the gate *before* it evokes pain perception and response (Melzack, 1982).

The Gate control theory, with its emphasis on a dynamic balance between excitory and inhibitory influences has been the basis of new approaches to pain therapy in all fields of medicine. It opens the way to understanding how the psychosociological make-up of individuals can influence their attitudes and reactions to pain; it also shows how certain movements can assist in pain reduction.

Nociceptive circuitry can be interfered with by:

- Transcutaneous electrical nerve stimulation (TENS) (see p. 216).
- Acupuncture (see p. 216).
- Chemical or pharmacological modulation.
- Mobilisation techniques in physiotherapy using mid-range, repetitive movements which stimulate the gate-closing sensory nerves.
- Any counter-irritant applied to the area of pain. Since time immemorial 'rubbing it better' has been man's intuitive method of using this theory (Bowsher, 1988b).

Back pain

The search for the cause of back pain would be simple if the fault could be laid at the door of one specific part, but there is rarely one source. Since the 1960s research into dead and living tissues has added to our knowledge of the intricacies of pain, the mechanics of joint movement, the role played by neural tissue, the process of injury and repair. One of the most revealing discoveries has been that *structural change* in itself need not give pain (McKenzie, 1981). A known condition like osteoarthritis is not necessarily the direct cause of pain. Pain arises only when the *function* of a sensitive tissue is compromised and altered for whatever reason (ibid).

Examination of the patient

The physiotherapist's approach to diagnosis or discovery of faulty function can only be achieved by careful assessment:

- Attention is paid to the patient's history of injury and pain, both past and present; old falls or whiplash injuries can give valuable clues; other pains present in the body which may not appear relevant can be vitally significant, for example, headaches in a patient with repetitive low back pain.
- The patient's occupation and social situation are relevant on two counts: first, to know what is happening to their body all day; second, to appreciate the psychosociological factors which may affect the course of recovery and which will determine the physiotherapist's approach.
- The patient is asked: Where is the pain? Does it vary in character? How long does it last? Is it constant or does it come and go? How does the pain respond to movement and to rest? The answers will provide essential clues.
- On examination the first need is to evaluate the patient's posture as a whole, and then the posture in relation to what the patient does all day, with a view to correcting any faults or difficulties.
- During the examination, which involves movement of the whole back and the relevant limbs, the physiotherapist is trying to elicit the patient's pain in a careful way, with respect for the irritability of the condition. If pain is acute the examination will have to be reduced

considerably. Everything is important: the reactions which provoke the pain, the positions which relieve it; the presence of restricted movement; the reaction of the muscles, joints and neural tissue to certain tests. A full neurological examination may be necessary if there are any signs of neural involvement. The physiotherapist is searching for detailed and precise responses of the body to movement which correspond to the patient's account of the pain. Treatment is based upon these findings.

The nature of back pain

Whether transient, acute or chronic, pain is a messenger of discomfort, and as such, it is the most revealing aid for diagnosis.

In an earlier example, you pulled your finger back as far as it would go until the base of it was really stinging. Do it again now, and hold it there for as long as you can. Keep holding it. The discomfort will eventually become pain and the pain will soon be so intense that you will have to let go. On release, the sting lasts for a few minutes, then recovers and the finger returns to normal. No damage has been done. The magnitude of pain is not always relative to the degree of damage caused. This was a transient pain. However, if you were forced to remain in that position for hours, or if you repeated the severe stretch over and over again, or if you bent it back violently and suddenly, beyond the point of tolerance, tissue damage would result; there would be acute pain of a much more persistent nature, possibly with redness, heat and swelling, giving pain every time you move the finger. Substitute the back for this example and it is possible to visualise the types of injury which can occur with the typical accompanying pain pattern.

Transient back pain can be the twinge of the over-stretch or the slightly awkward movement, a passing pain, but one which should not be ignored as it serves as a warning to avoid repetition.

Acute back pain can be either the acute pain which builds up from long sustained poor posture or long repeated stooping postural movements; or the acute pain following a sudden traumatic movement, one which lingers and disables in varying degrees. Both these acute pains warn that tissue damage has taken place, no matter how small, and the situation requires attention: attention first to heal the damage and reduce the pain, then to restore full function to the whole area. One of the worst lines of action is to 'soldier on', heroically persevering with all normal activities, trying to pretend the pain does not exist.

It is important to have a sense of proportion in relation to back pain. There is no need to be anxious over the first appearance but its messages must be respected and acted on. Sufferers must take responsibility for their actions, heeding the first pain warning which says 'don't repeat this, please' and putting back care into top priority; if not, injury will be reinforced and the period of disablement prolonged.

The chances for successful rehabilitation are reduced in patients in whom pain persists for more than six months. Even after three months of persistent pain the psychological make-up of the person may be altered (Nachemson, 1985). Chapter 17, p. 181, describes how to cope with an acute attack of back pain.

Chronic back pain: It is hypothesised that if acute pain was always fully resolved chronic pain would be minimised (Twomey and Taylor, 1987). Physiotherapists are trained never to 'assume' anything about pain (Maitland, 1986). Care must be taken not to discount a single sign or symptom expressed by the patient until the picture of the pain has been thoroughly and carefully examined, from both subjective and objective aspects. Although chronic pain may exist after all healing has taken place, clinicians must be very sure that this is actually the case and that their examination has not overlooked certain residual malfunctions (McCaffery, 1972); these are often sensed by the patient in their very understandable search for a solution. *The accuracy of this examination in itself must be carefully re-evaluated by every clinician* (Grieve, 1987).

Far too many chronic or long-term pain problems, classed as psychological or even 'psychogenic', have later been found to be complicated patterns of disorder. Examples of these are the 'chronic' symptoms of: whiplash injuries (Bogduk, 1986; Butler, 1991); cervical headache syndromes (Wells, 1988); conditions in which there is a large adverse neural tension component (Butler and Gifford, 1989), for example, coccydinia (Butler, 1991) and reflex sympathetic dystrophy (Butler, 1992); cervicobrachial pain syndromes (Elvey and Quintner, 1986; Boyling, 1991; Quintner, 1991; Cohen *et al.*, 1992); and of sympathetic maintained pain syndromes (Slater, 1991). Many of these conditions are now being dealt with successfully by treating all vertebral and peripheral structures involved, in particular the continuum of the nervous system and the interface through which it passes.

The chemical mediation of pain also plays a role in chronic low back pain. It has been found that the quantity of enkephalins and endorphins (morphine-like and opioid pain-reducing substances within the body) in the spinal nerve root and the cerebrospinal fluid, play an important role in the suppression of pain (Nachemson, 1985). Chronic back pain sufferers have a diminished amount of endorphins in the cerebrospinal fluid which is increased by activation of the large muscle groups (ibid). This provides food for thought for all rehabilitation.

Patients have often been driven to despair in the search for a solution to their pain, their depression being reinforced by misdiagnosis and the frustration of being disbelieved. When the lucky ones finally have their long-term pain relieved, the patients seem to shed the 'psychogenic' aura and become 'reasonable' human beings again (Watkins *et al.*, 1986).

The treatment of all chronic pain

Chronic incurable pain with no known cure is now being treated in many positive ways: **pain clinics** have been established in most major hospitals; **'schools for bravery'** exist (Aberg, 1984; Williams, 1989) in which sufferers are sympathetically guided, through physical and emotional rehabilitation towards the ability to live with their pain; **hospices** treat and comfort people with disabling pain from incurable diseases.

Cognitive techniques for pain control are being used as part of a more comprehensive programme to teach the relationship between thoughts, feelings, behaviour, environmental stimuli and pain. The procedures relate to the way patients perceive, interpret and relate to their pain rather than to the elimination of the pain *per se*, and this becomes the basis for therapy (Weisenberg, 1989). Self-appraisal is central to the method and the aim is for patients to be in control of their own pain (Craig, 1984).

Hypnosis and relaxation are being used successfully in the treatment of chronic pain. These techniques make use of the altered states of consciousness that are known to be attained through practices such as meditative prayer, transcendental meditation and autogenic therapy (Benson *et al.*, 1977). It is believed that in these states of consciousness a physiological response, termed the 'relaxation response', takes place which is distinctly different from that observed during quiet sitting or sleep, and involves changes consistent with decreased sympathetic nervous reaction (ibid).

The physiology of back pain

Knowledge of the mechanics of back pain is an essential requirement for understanding what may be occurring in a painful back.

Pain can arise from any pathological process that stimulates nociceptor endings (sensory receptors) in pain-sensitive structures of the back (Bogduk and Twomey, 1991); this means any tissue connected to or around the motion segment that has a nerve supply, including the innervated neural connective tissue.

Back pain varies in type depending on its cause. It can originate from a mechanical or chemical disturbance of tissue or a combination of both (McKenzie, 1981; Wyke, 1976). Pain can be experienced either locally, at the site of injury, or it can be referred into more distant areas.

Mechanical causes of back pain

Pain is produced by the application of mechanical forces as soon as the mechanical deformation of innervated structures is sufficient to irritate free nerve endings (McKenzie, 1981).

It can occur with or without tissue damage. With an absence of damage, the pain is merely from stressed tissues, followed by relief as soon as the stress is removed. The finger experiment is an example, as is low back pain which characteristically appears when sitting and disappears on standing (McKenzie, 1981). The pain can be caused by postural stress, stiff joint structures, locked or blocked joint structures, shortening of scarred tissue, even a minor disc bulge.

The nerve root, together with any pain sensitive structure within the vertebral canals or the IVF can be stretched, bent, or tethered at any point, eliciting pain. If the root is compromised for long, oedema can result which would lead to a chemical disturbance in the nerve tissue. Contrary to earlier belief, compression of the nerve root evokes paraesthesia and anaesthesia but not pain (Bogduk and Twomey, 1991).

Mechanical pain may be intermittent or constant, increased by certain positions and decreased by others or not, depending upon the ability to alter the deformation.

Chemical causes of back pain

Chemical pain is produced by chemical changes in the tissues which irritate the local nerve endings. It is caused by damage in trauma, infection, disease or ischaemia with resulting inflammation, swelling, increased heat, redness and tenderness, although these symptoms are not easily discernible in the back where the structures are hidden by layers of muscle. The pain is constant, unrelieved by any position, and often increased by movement.

Mechanical and chemical pain are both present in all trauma – strains, sprains, soft tissue lesions, disc lesions where there is extrusion of matter or wherever there is an inflammatory reaction.

Types of back pain

The source of pain may be mechanical or chemical but the sensation of pain can be experienced either locally or referred into other areas.

Local pain: somatic (body tissue) pain is a localised, mechanical or chemical disturbance of any of the pain-sensitive structures of the motion segments, including the muscles which are attached to or pass over them. The structures can be affected individually or in a combined way.

The pain is experienced at the site of the injury, the patient often being able to pinpoint the exact spot. The character of the pain depends on its mechanical or chemical origin.

Referred pain: referred pain is pain perceived in a region topographically displaced from the area that is the source of the pain (Bogduk, 1987). Not all low back pain is necessarily due to disorders of the lumbar spine. Lumbar pain may originate in visceral or vascular disease and this possibility must be assessed carefully on examination. Referred pain from the spine experienced in the limbs or trunk can be either **somatic** or **radicular**, (directly from a nerve root) in origin, but like all pain there must be a mechanical or chemical irritant.

Experiments in the past suggested that all referred pain followed a specific pattern into areas of the body but it has been found that referral from deep structures is not consistent from person to person (Hockaday and Whitty, 1967).

- **Somatic referred pain** is the mislocation of pain. The reasons for it are not clearly understood but is believed to stem from a misinterpretation of impulses received in the CNS from the tissues; pain that is generated by lesions in the spine may be perceived as emanating from the limbs or trunk. The mechanism appears to be that afferent (sensory) impulses from affected vertebral structures activate neurones in the CNS which also receive impulses from afferents in the limbs or other areas and the perception of these messages becomes confused (Bogduk and Twomey, 1991).

  Somatic referred pain can originate in any of the spinal structures, especially the disc or the Z joints. The pain is deep, vague and aching. The distance of referral is usually relative to the intensity of spinal stimulus (Mooney and Robertson, 1976; Bogduk, 1987); this relationship becomes very evident during the recovery of referred pain of this nature – as the condition improves the pain centralises, withdrawing towards the vertebral source of pain (McKenzie, 1981).

- **Radicular referred pain** originates from mechanical stimulation or traction of clinically damaged nerve roots or the dorsal root ganglia in the IVF (Bogduk and Twomey, 1991). The pain is a shooting, lancing type, often all the way down the limb in a specific line.

Compression of an undamaged nerve elicits paraesthesia and anaesthesia only. However, as it is impossible to say when a sound compressed nerve root may becomes a damaged nerve root. Any nerve deformation can eventually give rise to pain of radicular nature together with altered sensation, weakness of muscle and pins and needles (Bogduk and Twomey, 1991).

Pain is becoming less of a mystery as research investigates its mechanisms but the involved interconnections between psyche (the soul) and soma (the body) still present many fascinating unsolved problems.

Cohen *et al.*, (1992) sum up with a chronic pain paradigm which identifies three levels of contributing factors: nociceptive, neuropathic and psychogenic:

- The nociceptive level is familiar as that of tissue disease or damage; however, nociception strictly refers to the signalling of tissue damage or the threat thereof and may reflect altered function as well as altered structure.
- Defining a neuropathic level acknowledges that between the soma and the psyche is interposed the nervous system, itself a plastic structure, the function of which may change in response to afferent barrage.
- The psychogenic level acknowledges that the behavioural expression of pain depends on the interaction of the organism with its past experience, culture and environment.

The approach of clinicians, therapists, nurses and carers is summarised by Porter (1986) who says that we need to listen, observe, record and learn from patients' experience in order to unravel the mystery of pain, and by Maitland (1986) who says, simply, we must listen, we must search, and we must believe.

On the practical level of everyday back care it is essential to 'think mechanically'; to become more aware of the reasons why we get aches and pains and to attempt to avoid provocation of these mechanically intricate, tough, yet potentially sensitive structures.

The next chapter on the process of injury and repair should help to make the timescale of back injury more understandable.

REFERENCES

Aberg, J. (1984). Evaluation of an advanced back pain rehabilitation program, *Spine*, **9**(3), 317–318.

Baxter, R. (1988). Neuropharmacology of the pain pathway. *Pain: Management and control in physiotherapy* (Wells, P., Frampton, V. and Bowsher, D. eds.) Heinemann Medical Books.

Beecher, H.K. (1959). *The Measurement of Subjective Responses*, Oxford University Press.

Benson, H., Kotch, J.B., Crassweller, K.D. and Greenwood, M.M. (1977). Historical and clinical considerations of the relaxation response, *American Scientist*, **65**, (July–August), 441–445.

Bogduk, N. (1986). The anatomy and pathophysiology of whiplash, *Clin. Biomech.*, **1**, 92–101.

Bogduk, N. (1987). Innervation, pain patterns, and mechanisms of pain production. *Physical Therapy of the Low Back*. (Twomey, L.T. and Taylor, J.R. eds.) Churchill Livingstone

Bogduk, N. and Twomey, L.T. (1991). *Clinical Anatomy of the Lumbar Spine*, 2nd ed., Churchill Livingstone, Singapore.
Bond, M.R. (1984). *Pain: its Nature, Analysis and Treatment*, 2nd ed., Churchill Livingstone.
Bowsher, D. (1988a). Acute and chronic pain and assessment, *Pain: Management and Control in Physiotherapy*, (Wells, P., Frampton, V. and Bowsher, D. eds.), Heinemann Medical Books.
Bowsher, D. (1988b). Modulation of nociceptive input, *Pain: Management and Control in Physiotherapy*, Wells, P., Frampton, V. and Bowsher, D. (eds.), Heinemann Medical Books.
Boyling, J. (1991). Upper limb disorders in the work place, OCPPP *In Touch*, Autumn, **61**, 14–16.
Butler, D. (1991). *Mobilisation of the Nervous System*, Churchill Livingstone.
Butler, D. (1992) (personal communication). *Mobilisation of the Nervous System*, Lecture.
Butler, D. and Gifford, L. (1989). The concept of adverse mechanical tension in the nervous system, *Physiotherapy*, **75**(11), 622–635.
Carpenito, W. (1983). *Nursing Diagnosis: Application to Clinical Practice*, J.B. Lippincott Co., Philadelphia.
Cohen, M.L., Arroyo, J.F., Champion, G.D. and Browne, C.D. (1992). In search of the pathogenesis of refractory cervicobrachial pain syndromes, *Med. J. Aust.*, **156**(March), 16.
Craig, K.D. (1984). Emotional aspects of pain, *Textbook of Pain*, (Wall, P.D. and Melzack, R., eds.), Churchill Livingstone.
Egbert, L.D., Battit, G.E., Welch, C.E. and Bartlett, M.K. (1964). Reduction of postoperative pain by encouragement and instruction of patients, *N. Eng. J. Med.*, **270**(16), 825–827.
Elvey, R.L. and Quinter, J.L. (1986). A clinical study of RSI, *Australian Family Physician*, **15**(10).
Fabrega, H. and Tyma, S. (1976). Language and cultural influences in the description of pain. *Br. J. Med. Psychol.*, **49**, 349–371.
Fields, H.L. and Basbaum, A. (1984). Endogenous pain control mechanisms, *Textbook of Pain*, (Wall, P.D. and Melzack, R., eds.), Churchill Livingstone.
Fordham, M. (1992). Pain, *Patient Problems* (Wilson-Barnett, J. and Batehup, L., eds.), Scutari Press.
French, S. (1989). Pain: Some psychological and sociological aspects, *Physiotherapy*, **75**(5).
Grieve, G.P. (1987). Some psychological aspects of benign spinal pain, *Physiotherapy*, **73**(9), 499–501.
Hardy, J.D., Wolff, H.G. and Goodell, H. (1952). *Pain Sensations and Reactions*, Williams and Wilkins, Baltimore.
Hayward, J. (1981). Information – a prescription against pain, *Royal College of Nursing of the United Kingdom*, **2**(6).
Hockaday, J.M. and Whitty, C.W.M. (1967). Patterns of referred pain in the normal subject, *Brain*, **90**(3), 481–495.
International Association for the Study of Pain (1979). Sub-committee on taxonomy, *Pain*, **6**, 249–252
Leriche, R. (1939). *The Surgery of Pain*. Williams and Wilkins, Baltimore.
Maitland, G.D. (1986). *Vertebral Manipulation*, 5th ed., Butterworths.
McCaffery, M. (1972). *Nursing Management of the Patient with Pain*, J.B. Lippincott, Philadelphia.
McKenzie, R. (1981). *The Lumbar Spine and Mechanical Diagnosis*, Spinal Publications.
Melzack, R. (1982). Recent concepts of pain, *Journal of Medicine*, **13** (3), 147–160.
Melzack, R. and Wall, P. (1965). Pain mechanisms: a new theory, *Science*, **150**(3699).

Melzack, R. and Wall, P. (1991). *The Challenge of Pain*, revised ed., Penguin Books.

Mooney, V. and Robertson, J. (1976). The facet syndrome. *Clin. Orthop.*, **115**, March–April, 149–156.

Nachemson, A. (1985). Recent advances in the treatment of low back pain, *International Orthopaedics* (SICOT), **9**, 1–10.

Pavlov, I.P. (1927). *Conditioned Reflexes*, (Anrep, G.V., ed. and tr.), Oxford University Press.

Porter, R.W. (1986). *Management of Back Pain*, Churchill Livingstone.

Quintner, J. (1991). The RSI syndrome in historical perspective, *Int. Disabil. Studies*, **13**, 99–103.

Slater, H. (1991). Adverse neural tension in the sympathetic trunk and sympathetic maintained syndromes, *7th biennial conference proceedings: Manipulative Physiotherapists Association of Australia*, 214–218.

Sternbach, R.A. and Tursky, B. (1965). Ethnic differences among housewives in psychophysical and skin potential responses to electric shock, *Psychophysiology*, **1**(3).

Sternbach, R.A. (1989). Acute versus chronic pain, *Textbook of Pain*, (Wall, P. and Melzack, R., eds.), 2nd ed., Churchill Livingstone.

Twomey, L.T. and Taylor, J.R. (1987). The lumbar spine, low back pain and physical therapy, *Physical Therapy of the Low Back*, (Twomey, L.T. and Taylor, J.R., eds.), Churchill Livingstone.

Watkins, R.G., O'Brien, J.P., Draugelis, R. and Jones, D. (1986). Comparisons of pre-operative & post-operative MMPI data in chronic back pain patients. *Spine*, **11**, 385.

Weisenberg, M. (1989). Cognitive aspects of pain, *Textbook of Pain*, (Wall, P. and Melzack, R., eds.), 2nd Ed., Churchill Livingstone.

Wells, P. (1988). Introduction, *Pain: Management and Control in Physiotherapy*, (Wells, P., Frampton, V. and Bowsher, D., eds.), Heinemann Medical Books.

Williams, J.I. (1989). Illness behaviour to wellness behaviour: the school for bravery approach, *Physiotherapy*, **75**(1), 2–7.

Wyke, B. (1976). Neurological aspects of low back pain, *The Lumbar Spine and Back Pain*, (Jayson, M.I.V., ed.), Pitman Publishing.

Zborowski, M. (1952). Cultural components in response to pain, *Journal of Sociological Issues* **8**, 16.

Zborowski, M. (1969). *People in Pain*, Jossey-Bass Inc., San Francisco.

8. *Injury*

The process of injury and healing

Impatience with illness and injury is a healthy and natural reaction. Most people long to return to normal living, and are often bewildered by the strange, uncontrollable forces which dominate their bodies. They are uncertain about the best way to handle the pain, afraid of doing something that makes things worse and frustratedbecause the injury 'should be better by now'. As a result, they either avoid movement altogether, which leads to stiffness and later trouble, or they struggle on in spite of pain, trying to function 'normally' – which frequently continues to irritate and prolong the injurious process. Understanding the timescale involved in the process of injury and healing removes both fear and frustration. Healing cannot be accelerated but correct handling can avoid the delay caused by repeated injury and so make recovery faster (Evans, 1980).

The process described takes place in any soft tissue trauma. It does not include open wound healing or care which are covered in detail by Torrance (1986) and Westaby (1985).

The process of injury and healing takes place in three stages: injury, inflammation and repair:

Injury: during the course of any soft tissue injury, a sprain, bruise or crush, the local network of blood vessels is damaged; some of the tissues are deprived of blood supply and so the cells die (Evans, 1980). Fibrous tissue in the area may also be structurally damaged and so within a few minutes of injury the area contains a collection of dead and dying tissue cells (ibid). A series of chemical changes then take place. The dying cells break down and release chemicals which affect other nearby cells and capillaries, causing the blood vessels to become more permeable. The blood vessels release blood which contains dead red cells, dead platelets and plasma. The platelets in turn release thrombin, an enzyme, which turns one of the plasma proteins (fibrinogen) into fibrin. Fibrin forms a network of fibres, enmeshing the debris of dead cells into a blood clot (ibid). The area begins to feel sore, stiff and achy and the next phase, inflammation, has started.

Inflammation: the four signs of inflammation are calor (heat), rubor (redness), dolor (pain) and tumor (swelling).

- **Heat and redness.** Immediately after injury there is a brief vasoconstriction in the area soon followed by dilation of the blood vessels as a result of chemical action and the axon reflex of arterioles (Thomson *et al.*, 1991). The area is flooded with blood and becomes pink and warm. Change of colour may never be noticeable in the back due to the quantity of muscle bulk between the injury and the skin, but heat is palpable.
- **Pain.** All the chemicals released into the tissue fluids bathe the nerve endings causing a further release of chemicals, with the resulting increase of pain (Melzack and Wall, 1991).
- **Swelling.** Swelling only occurs immediately if there is substantial bleeding, otherwise it takes a few hours to manifest. Four hours after the injury, white cells begin to migrate through the vessel walls into the damaged area to start their job of scavenging and devouring the debris. The area now contains a mass of inflammatory exudate, the pressure of which further irritates nerve endings, enhancing the pain. *The inflammatory exudate may still be increasing for three to five days depending upon the severity of the injury or the amount of re-injury inflicted* (Evans, 1980).

Repair: finally, on the third to fifth day the process of repair begins, a process that lasts approximately six weeks. It starts when nearby cells begin to divide and multiply. While the exudate is gradually being removed by the white cells, new capillaries bud and grow in from the perimeter of the debris, bringing fresh oxygen. Fibroblast cells start to lay down fibrils of collagen in the exudate which grow to become bundles of collagen or fibrous tissue, and healing takes place. The larger the quantity of exudate, the greater the amount of fibrous tissue. In other words, *the quantity of scar tissue depends upon the amount of swelling*.

Healed tissue is never the same as it was before, it is replaced but it never has quite the same structure or properties as the original (Evans, 1980; Torrance, 1986). Scar tissue has the property of gradually shortening when it is fully formed, a process which occurs from the third week to the sixth month after injury (Evans, 1980).

From this timescale three clear, linked guidelines emerge for the treatment of injury:

- Try to reduce swelling as much as possible and so avoid massive scar tissue.
- Respect the injury for at least three to five days and avoid provocation for six weeks.
- Gradually but steadily restore normal movement, ensuring full-range mobility with no restrictions on previous range.

Ignoring the injury period by allowing repeated damage and increased exudate to develop not only lengthens the time of healing but inevitably leads to increased scar formation and loss of previous movement range.

Injury and back pain

The approach to back pain should be that of the sleuth searching for vital clues. The first sign of trouble should initiate the question, 'What has provoked this?' or 'What happened yesterday?' or 'Have my activities this week been different from usual?' Assessment of the cause of injury can assist diagnosis and help to avoid further aggravation.

It can be difficult: apparently innocent situations like a twinge of back pain while decorating followed by a long car drive at the weekend could well be a trigger; or an evening spent sitting in the theatre after a heavy day's work and a fast game of squash could be a reason for waking the next morning unable to move.

Discovering the aggravating factor can provide the danger position to avoid and recognising the sequence of events gives an intimation as to how much provocation the back can take. This information is invaluable for future back care.

After any trauma, if pain is disabling or unrelenting, if there is any degree of referred pain or disturbing symptoms such as loss of sensation, paraesthesia or muscle weakness a doctor should be consulted.

Providing there are no untoward complications, the reduction of swelling is the first aim; ice, rest and possibly anti-inflammatory drugs are the three immediate treatments (see How to cope with an acute attack, Chapter 17, p. 181, where ice application is covered in more detail).

Rest

The quantity of rest required depends on the degree of injury and the severity of pain. It can vary from merely taking care by avoiding provocative movements to implementing complete bed rest.

The benefits of bed rest have received considerable investigation recently and it appears to be clear that prolonged rest is actually deleterious, especially in relation to chronic pain (Deyo *et al.*, 1986; Nachemson, 1983; Twomey and Taylor, 1991). Protracted rest leads to a catabolic state with general malaise, eventually leading to demineralisation of bone and 3 per cent loss of muscle per day (Waddell, 1989). Deyo's (1986) research found that two days' bed rest was as beneficial as seven in cases of straightforward low back pain without any discogenic or pain referral complications.

Research into joint reaction to pain shows that:

- Mid-range gentle movements actually reduce pain (Williams and Sperryn, 1979; Maitland, 1986).
- Movement improves the nutrition of all structures of the motion segment (discussed earlier).
- Activation of large muscle groups increases the level of endorphins in cerebrospinal fluid, which in turn reduces levels of pain sensitivity (Nachemson, 1985) (see Chapter 7, p. 94).

So gentle movements within the limits of pain actually reduce pain and enhance the healing process, 'within the limits of pain' being the important factor: pain means provocation which in turn means re-injury. It is clear that total inactivity is not advantageous except when used within the prime aim of reducing the inflammatory reaction in those first crucial days.

The criteria for rest in acute pain must be based upon the severity of symptoms and the early relief of pain:

- It is best to continue living reasonably normally with careful avoidance of provocative activity – providing that pain allows it, that back care is implemented fully, and that obvious daily improvement is achieved.
- However, if there is unmistakable deterioration; with symptoms such that no relief can be found in any upright position; or if leg pain is present, then bed rest is the only answer.

'Bed rest' must be *complete rest*, either in bed or on the floor, whichever gives greater relief. It does *not* mean slouching on the sitting room sofa craning the neck round in a distorted twist to watch TV, nor does it mean reading propped up in bed on a pile of cushions with the lumbar spine flexed and both legs straight out in front. Rest that is inadequate is worse than careful activity because it makes the sufferer feel he/she is resting while the injury is probably being provoked further: 'I've rested for a whole week and my pain is still as bad as ever!'

The body should be completely supported horizontally, relaxed in any position, lying supine, prone or on the side, with frequent changes of position (see Chapter 17, p. 182). Any position which reduces pain should be adopted for at least five minutes every hour, any position which increases pain should be avoided.

Anti-inflammatory medication

Cortisol, the most active steroid derivative, is extremely effective in reducing the inflammatory effect when injected into the site in the first three or four days after injury, but there are reservations about its effect on the healing process (Evans, 1980). Non-steroidal anti-inflammatory drugs (NSAIDs), of which there are many, have three therapeutic actions: against pain, against inflammation and against fever (Melzack and Wall, 1991). Some react directly upon the tissues and some via the nervous system. They are of value during an inflammatory reaction. In certain cases, however, anti-inflammatory drugs are contraindicated for 48 hours after injury as they can delay the clotting process.

Recovery

After the first three to five days, those who have been resting should be up and those who have been continuing with careful activity should be becoming gradually more pain-free. If not, a doctor should be consulted.

The repair process should now be aided by gently increasing movement without re-traumatising until a fully pain-free situation is achieved (see Chapter 17, p. 186).

The average back injury takes six weeks to recover and in severe cases can take six months or a year. The return to full function and full range activity means diligent but careful stretching throughout this time (Evans, 1980).

Emotional recovery from back pain is as important as physical recuperation. It is essential for the sufferer to feel that he or she has 'got over' the injury, and that there is no longer a 'weakness'. While uncertainty exists, there will be vulnerability which will lead to re-injury.

REFERENCES

Deyo, R.A., Diehl, A.K., Rosenthal, M. (1986). How many days of bed rest for acute low back pain? *N. Engl. J. Med.*, **October 23**, 1064–1070.

Evans, P. (1980). The healing process at cellular level: a review, *Physiotherapy*, **66**(8), 256–259.

Maitland, G.D. (1986). *Vertebral Manipulation*, 5th ed., Butterworths.

Melzack, R. and Wall, P. (1991). *The Challenge of Pain*, Revised ed., Penguin Books.

Nachemson, A. (1983). Work for all: for those with low back pain as well, *Clin. Orthop.*, **179**, 77–85.

Nachemson, A. (1985). Recent advances in the treatment of low back pain, *International Orthopaedics* (SICOT) **9**, 1–10.

Thomson, A., Skinner, A. and Piercy, J. (1991). *Tidy's Physiotherapy*, 12th ed., Butterworths.

Torrance, C. (1986). The physiology of wound healing, *Nursing*, **5**, 162–168.

Twomey, L.T. and Taylor, J.R. (1991). age-related changes of the lumbar spine and spinal rehabilitation, reprinted from the CRC Critical Reviews in *Physical and Rehabilitation Medicine*, **2**(3), 153–169, CRC Press, Inc.

Waddell, G. (1989). A new clinical model for the treatment of low back pain, *Back Pain. New Approaches to Rehabilitation and Education* (Roland, M. and Jenner, J.R. eds.), Manchester University Press.

Westaby, S. (ed.) (1985). *Wound Care*, Heinemann Medical Books.

Williams, J.G.P. and Sperryn, P.N. (1979). *Sports Medicine*, Edward Arnold, London.

9. Causes of back pain

There is no one source of back pain but the causes can be divided into **predisposing** (indirect) and **precipitating** (direct) factors (McKenzie, 1981). Predisposing factors cause an insidious, ever-growing stress on the structures of the back, creating a vulnerability which can, with minor provocation, escalate into a full-blown episode of severe pain. They are:

- Postural abuse.
- Prolonged lumbar flexion.
- Loss of mobility.
- Work-related stress.
- Obesity.
- Debilitating conditions.

Precipitating factors are either the 'last straw' or are in themselves immediate instigators of tissue trauma. They can be classed under the headings coined by Maitland (1986):

- New use.
- Misuse.
- Overuse.
- Ebuse, (trauma).

Predisposing factors

Postural abuse

Poor standing posture: the variety of different postures is profuse. Some types increase certain curves, others decrease them. However, allowing for slight variation in skeletal type, there is only one prototype posture (see Chapter 11, p. 121). Most poor postures tend to slump in one way or another, sagging, losing muscle tone, hanging on the hip and spinal ligaments, mistreating and stressing all the structures in and around the motion segment – a breeding ground for back pain.

Static posture is provocative, especially when fixed, asymmetric and awkward (Boyling, 1992); many occupational stances entail working with machinery which requires a distorted body posture maintained without respite for hours. This can lead to postural deformity which in time, if uncorrected, can elicit considerable pain.

Computer workers function with static vertebral postures (often maintained with tension around the shoulder area), an awkward head position and hands that are held fixed on the keyboard – only the fingers move. Patients frequently ascribe shoulder pain acquired under these conditions to 'tension', possibly because they are under a certain amount of office pressure – but they forget to examine and analyse their work-related posture. For example, they may sit with the keyboard on their left and the computer screen on their right so that the head spends most of the day in a rotated position; added to this, the screen can be too high or too low, causing further mechanical stress to their already rotated cervical Z Joints (see Chapter 15, p. 163).

Adolescent postures: during the growth spurts in human development, the first between the ages of 6 and 8 years and the second between 12 and 16, bone grows faster than soft tissue. Muscles and ligaments lag behind the bone length by about 6– 8 months and so does the neural tissue. This leads to tightness of tissues, especially those of the limbs, with considerable adverse neural tension (Butler, 1992). Headaches, knee problems, calf pain and poor posture can all result.

In an attempt to cover up their breast growth, adolescent girls sometimes develop a thoracic kyphosis with a poking chin posture in which the head is held in greater extension compared with the flexed lower cervical spine. In the cervical spine the sympathetic trunk is situated anterior to the transverse processes and is therefore placed on stretch in head extension positions. In the poking chin posture undue tension is exerted continuously on the sympathetic trunk; possibly causing symptoms of nausea, vague thoracic pains and headaches (Butler, 1991). This applies, of course, to all such postures.

Prolonged lumbar flexion

The lumbar lordosis is the natural lumbar curve. The size of the curve varies in degree with different skeletal characteristics. There is no evidence that a lesser lordosis is less beneficial than a larger curve, providing that the curve, which is structurally important to the resilience and spring of the vertebral column, is maintained without adverse postural stress. It is the loss of the 'natural' lordosis that becomes injurious. The natural curve is altered by continuous poor posture and constant repetition of postural situations where the lumbar spine is maintained in flexion.

The most injurious positions are:

- **Poor sitting postures** in which the lumbar spine is forced into a more flexed attitude with the pelvis allowed to tip back on flexed hips and the whole spine is rounded into a C-shape. The cervical spine, unable to stay comfortably upright, droops into a 'poking chin' posture. The weight of the arms, head and thorax tends to be thrust into the stretched soft tissues of the lower back. Sitting becomes a hazard in all sedentary desk occupations, in driving, in certain specialist jobs that involve looking down, such as dentistry – or while slouching in a chair watching television.

- **Prolonged stooping** which provides another sustained position in flexion, often involving outstretched arms with heavy objects in the hands. Bending forwards in this way is part of most standing occupations such as nursing, certain manufacturing stances, manual activities, household chores and anything to do with children. It places endless strain on all portions of the motion segment (see Chapter 4, p. 44).
- **Repetitive bending.** Closely related to prolonged stooping, repetitive bending involves a constant up-and-down action, often holding a weight in the hands, never or rarely resuming the true upright position and so never restoring the lordosis. It occurs in many occupations, for example, building or road work, gardening, nursing, housework, and industrial packaging. Lifting added to repetitive bending ensures an even greater vulnerability to sudden stress or trauma.

Loss of mobility

Loss of mobility can result from lack of use or poor recovery from injury.

Lack of use: a decrease in the range of movement of the spine potentially reduces its response to sudden demand, the stiff and inelastic tissues being unable to yield or accommodate to the extra requirement. Prolonged inactivity of any kind leads to muscle atrophy, loss of strength and adaptive shortening of soft tissue (Taylor and Twomey,1987). Research provides evidence that inactivity actually hinders cartilage and soft tissue repair whereas repetitive passive or mid-range movement accelerates regeneration and stimulates the activity of synovial fluid within joints (Evans, 1980;Salter, 1975;Williams and Sperryn, 1979).

Poor recovery from episodes of back pain, in which there has been some lumbar kyphosis due to muscle spasm, can lead to a loss of mobility. Restoration of the natural lordosis with a regime of active exercises and postural correction is an essential part of recovery.

All of this underlines the need to maintain full range joint mobility. Full range means the whole extent of possible movement from the fully-flexed position to the fully-extended position, from the fully-rotated position one way to the fully-rotated position in the other direction, likewise with side bending (see **1.1**, p. 10). It is important to realise that flexion of the spine as an exercise is not an abuse, it needs to be performed as well as any other movement. The spine need not be exercised energetically every day to maintain mobility. A few precise movements in all directions are sufficient, providing the movement is taken up to the end of range and nudged further to stretch it slightly. Fast repetitive movements facilitate muscle strengthening or aerobic stimulation, but they do not accomplish maintenance of range.

The most valuable aid to preserving full body movement is **physical awareness**, being able to feel how the body moves, being able to sense the restrictions within it and then knowing how to encourage movement into and beyond those limits, gently but firmly.

Mobility of the hips and knees plays a fundamental role in back care. Weak quadriceps muscles (see **5.1**, p. 62) prohibit rising from the squat position; if squatting is impossible, the correct techniques of lifting can never be mastered and stooping will be inevitable when retrieving something from the floor. Weakness and immobility of the hips and knees advances insidiously with age unless a concerted effort is made to counteract it. Exercising is one way but conscious attention to daily habits can play a vital role.

How many times a day do you use your arms instead of your leg muscles? What do you do when you bend down to reach something in a low cupboard? Instead of using your legs to stand upright again, you put your hands on the work top or other handy surface and heave yourself up. What do you do when you rise from a chair? You put your hands on the arm of the chair and push yourself up instead of moving to the front of the chair and forcing your legs to work on their own. What happens when you climb the stairs? You hang on to the banisters, pulling with one arm, again decreasing the amount of work done by the leg muscles. Hold on to the banisters for safety, but do not use them to assist leg activity. Every time you avoid one of these actions you are losing the opportunity of working muscles naturally and keeping them up to strength. Weak muscles leave joints unprotected and more susceptible to the slightest injury.

Work-related stress conditions

Force and vibration: force and vibration inflicted on the body by any tools, by the use of your hands or by materials can cause unnatural stresses, especially around the neck and shoulders for example: pneumatic drills, constant hammering, wearing heavy gloves (Boyling, 1992). All driving, especially of heavy vehicles such as tractors, gives a vibration stress which may affect the axial loading of the discs (Anderson, 1987).

Frequency and duration of work: in industrial occupations there is often too great a force required to perform a job with too little time to relax in order to recuperate. The problems are related to the skill and confidence of the performer, the performer's age in relation to the magnitude of the task and, not least, to the financial element whereby stress is provoked by the demand for increased productivity (Boyling, 1992).

Obesity

Excessive weight is a common problem and a notoriously difficult one to overcome. Apart from appearance, which is a matter of opinion, the strain on the heart and the tendency towards high blood pressure are well-known complications. The effect upon the back, however, is not immediately recognisable, even less so, perhaps, than the effect on the hips and knees.

The most common consequence for the back is an increased lordosis brought about by the bulk of the abdomen so that the lumbar spine is dragged forwards into hyperextension. This is a familiar condition of pregnancy, often with resulting back pain, but pregnancy comes to an end and the spine can return to normal.

Wear and tear is the final outcome of the stress on all joints with an increased lordosis. The lumbar Z joints can finally become impacted in extension, and osteoarthritis can develop prematurely in the Z joints, the hips and knees, leading to loss of mobility everywhere.

Loss of mobility is a covert companion to obesity. No matter how apparently mobile the obese person's joints remain, all tissue bulk obstructs full movement of any joint, whether the back, the hips or the knees, and the joints can never be put through their full range.

Dieting is a complicated problem for many, as it is so tied up with inner needs and desires. Professional help should be sought if self-restraint is impossible. In any situation, a weight problem is best discussed with a doctor before starting a dietary regime.

Debilitating conditions

Chemical changes which take place in joints during any inflammatory state have already been discussed. During or immediately after any viral infection, any systemic condition or any local joint inflammation, especially during the period of recuperation, considerable care should be taken of the back in all situations, avoiding any possible risk or stress.

Precipitating factors

Precipitating factors are the direct and sudden causes of back pain. They can provoke a previously pain-free back or they can trigger an abused back which has a history of previous trouble

New use

Any previously unperformed and unpractised activity can be structurally provocative; so can a movement that has not been performed for some time, if it is done for too long or too strenuously or beyond the capabilities of structures involved, at their present state of health. There are many examples: taking on a lifting job after a previously sedentary occupation, digging a new garden after years of living in a flat, playing a strenuous game of squash for the first time in middle age.

Misuse

Awkward movements: injury can occur at any moment when concentration is sufficiently diminished to allow a minute loss of co-ordination or when an activity is carried out in an awkward manner: bending to pick up a thread from the carpet, reaching sideways to turn out the light, stretching upwards into a cupboard. These are all normal movements which if performed correctly would cause no ill-effect but with muscular imbalance, or sudden movement, tissues can be quite severely stressed. A young healthy back might cope with these situations but a back that has suffered the trials of life often capitulates.

Awkward objects: lifting is always a hazard, even for a back free from all previous symptoms. As a cause of back pain, it is classed here as a misuse because if a manageable weight is lifted correctly there should be no resulting trauma. No matter how light the object, an incorrect lift can precipitate a problem; no matter how thorough the technique, if the load is too heavy, the potential for injury is great. It is therefore important to learn to lift correctly early in life and take every opportunity to practise making the correct movements habitual rather than a conscious effort. (see Chapter 14, p. 147).

Overuse

Overuse is very much the 'last straw'. On top of the accumulative effects of normal use – the odd niggling pain, an excessively tired body – overuse, stresses structures beyond their ability to adapt to demands and tissue injury occurs accompanied by severe pain.

Abuse (trauma)

Back injury can occur in any accident or violent movement when the body hits an object, is hit by something, or moves or falls in a sudden, uncontrolled manner. Nothing can prevent damage in these circumstances. Depending upon the severity of the trauma, injury can vary from tissue bruising to tissue sprain, to rupture of ligamentous or muscular structure, to bone fracture, end plate fracture, Z joint cartilage damage or intervertebral disc damage. In this situation a stiff back will tend to suffer greater injury than a healthy one undergoing an identical assault.

Coughing and sneezing: everyone who has experienced acute back pain will know how painful a cough or sneeze can be. The increase of pain comes partly from the sudden muscular movement jerking the back into flexion and partly because the enforced rib and abdominal compression increases the intra-abdominal pressure which in turn pressurises the sensitive structures in and around the vertebrae. However, a sudden, violent sneeze can actually precipitate a back problem. It is possible to reduce the risk by bracing the back and abdominal muscles firmly before the sneeze arrives and by bending both knees at the moment of impact.

Risk situations

By linking the predisposing and precipitating factors together in a practical sense certain risk situations emerge, some of them quite surprising moments in everyday living. These apparently innocuous situations can be the instantaneous cause of back injury.

Lifting after sitting for prolonged periods

Lifting after prolonged periods of sitting puts the back into a most vulnerable position. It is one of the more common holiday accidents. Holidays inevitably commence with a long journey sitting in a car, train, bus or aircraft. During this time the lumbar ligaments are stretched in flexion and the structures motionless, rarely moved even by alteration of position. At the end of the journey, invariably while still in a stooping posture, heavy suitcases are manhandled from the boot of the car or from the airport luggage collection carousel – and the damage is done. Pain need not manifest immediately, it can appear at any time from that moment to later the same day to first thing the next morning.

The answer is quite simple and will be stressed in Part 2 of this book – it is essential to restore the lordosis by arching the back as shown in **9.1** as soon as you rise from a sitting position. The longer the sitting posture has been maintained the more important it is to achieve the natural lordosis, even if the back feels a bit stiff trying to correct it. If this restoration is made, it is possible to lift carefully in greater safety.

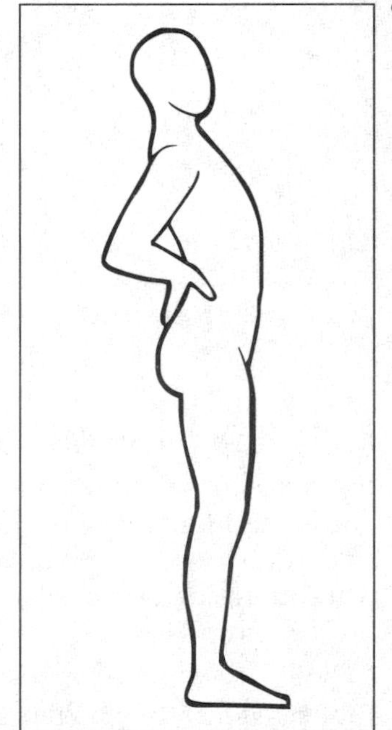

9.1 The routine back arch after sitting or stooping

Slouching after vigorous exercise

This is rather a surprising danger, and it catches out sports people all too frequently. After a day's hard work, a game of squash seems to be an ideal relaxation. However, having exhausted all the muscles with energetic activity, warmed up and tired all the back structures, the worst possible position to adopt is total relaxation in a big floppy armchair – even more so after a hot bath. The tissues allow themselves to be stretched into flexion without complaint, giving no warning of the stress taking place until the next morning, when getting out of bed can be almost impossible. So often the thought is 'I must have done something to my back playing squash yesterday,' with little realisation that the damage was brought about by the mode of relaxation afterwards. The best relaxation after any strenuous activity is to lie supine or prone (preferably prone if comfortable) for 10–15 minutes. Lying supine on the floor with both lower legs on a chair is another possibility (**9.2**). Always restore the lordosis on standing after resting.

9.2

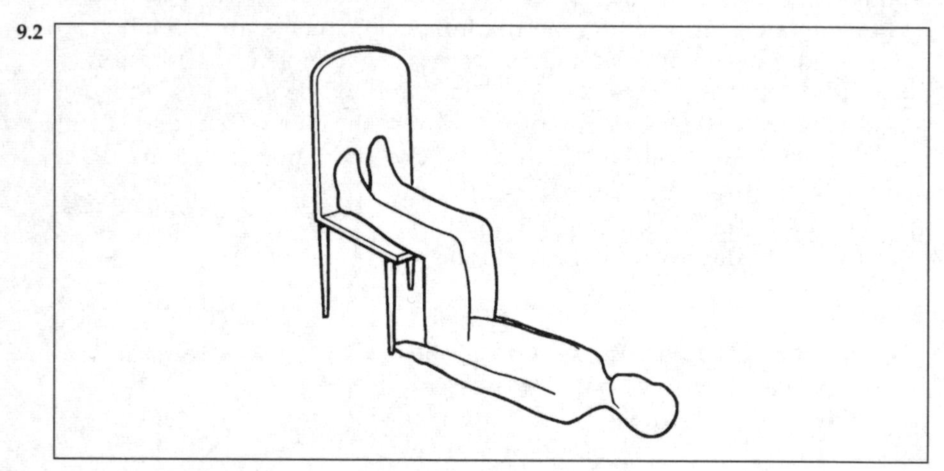

9.2 Recovery position for an aching back

Reaching up or stretching

Reaching up or stretching is frequently an off-balance position with the body weight more on one leg than the other. One side of the spine is concave while the other is convex, and in this precarious pose a slight twitch, extra stretch or loss of balance can tweak the back into trouble.

Prolonged standing

Prolonged standing becomes a risk because of the element of fatigue which causes slumping into the supportive ligaments. Maintaining good posture over a prolonged period requires concentration and frequent, nagging correction. It is not easy to maintain. For this reason, slow shopping expeditions are one of the most re-traumatising experiences for those people recovering from back pain.

Prolonged standing can be one of the rare extension stresses, depending upon the individual postural type. The rest position for pain caused by sustained extension stress in standing can be to curl up into flexion (**9.3**).

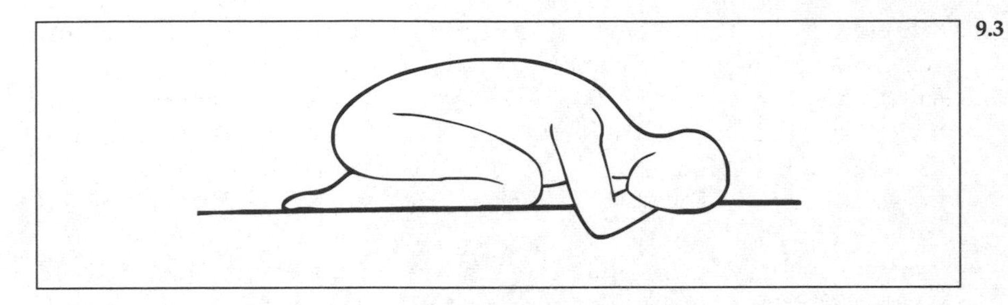

9.3

Part 1 of this book has been concerned with the kinds of damage sustainable in the human back. It must now be clear that diagnosis is impossible without individual and specialised investigations. A 'strained back' covers a multitude of possible injuries from a muscular strain to a Z joint malfunction, from postural abuse to a bulging disc. Fortunately, back care follows the same guidelines for most of these conditions – it relates to the functional signs and symptoms rather than the clinical or pathophysiological diagnosis.

REFERENCES

Anderson, J.A.D. (1987) Back pain and occupation, *The Lumbar Spine and Back Pain*, (Jayson, M.I.V., ed.), 3rd ed., Churchill Livingstone.
Boyling, J. (1992) (personal communication). *Repetitive Strain Injury*.
Butler, D. (1991). *Mobilisation of the Nervous System*, Churchill Livingstone.
Butler, D. (1992) (personal communication). Lecture course on *Mobilisation of the Nervous System*.
Evans, P. (1980). The healing process at cellular level, *Physiotherapy*, **66**(8).
Maitland, G.D. (1986). *Vertebral Manipulation*, 5th ed., Butterworths.
McKenzie, R. (1981). *The Lumbar Spine: Mechanical Diagnosis and Therapy*, Spinal Publications.
Salter, R.B., Simmonds, D.F. and Malcolm, B.W. (1975). Effects of continuous passive motion on the healing of articular cartilage defects. *J. Bone Joint Surg.*, **57A**(4), 570.
Taylor, J. and Twomey, L.T. (1987). The lumbar spine, low back pain and physical therapy, *Physical Therapy of the Low Back*, (Twomey, L.T. and Taylor J. eds.), Churchill Livingstone, USA.
Williams, J.G.P. and Sperryn P.N. (1979). *Sports Medicine*, Edward Arnold, London.

Part 2

Back care

10. *Prevention*

Postural care

Back care requires a knowledge about back structure, an awareness of potential injury and a resolve to prevent any detrimental occurrences. The first two have been covered in Part 1 – now we look at the prevention of injury and the prevention of further injury.

Injury can result from sudden trauma or from gradual deterioration associated with continuing abuse.

Trauma, such as injury from incorrect lifting, can be avoided by training and care, but accident is unavoidable. However, a healthy, mobile back will withstand trauma more readily than a stiff and thus vulnerable one.

Deterioration progresses in stages. Pain escalates from one step to another as abuse continues, often with shorter and shorter time between the stages. However, the process can be halted at any point by taking corrective measures, and the journey back to normality can be achieved with return to full functional movement:

- Poor posture...leads to stress on joints...leads to *pain* .
- Stress on joints...leads to joint malfunction...leads to *pain.*
- Joint malfunction...leads to distortion of disc and tissue...leads to *pain.*
- Distortion of disc and tissue...leads to disc bulge...leads to *pain* .

Prevention encompasses all postural care, whether standing, sitting, lying, working, lifting, carrying, pulling or pushing.

Chambers Dictionary defines 'posture' as 'the relative disposition of parts of the body'. Whatever the posture adopted, the relationship between one body part and the other is salient. Postural correction requires:

- Postural awareness, in ourselves and in others.
- A physical sensitivity to the contrast between tension and relaxation.
- An understanding of the varied purpose of specific exercise.

Positive critical evaluation goes hand in hand with growing awareness; comparison, when used constructively, is the best informer. Become an avid analyst of other people's movements; look with new eyes at every stance on television, at every slouch in the supermarket queue, at every walk strolling by the window. Having observed, then feel. The sensations of posture need to be perceived from within. To begin with, you may need mirrors to see the postures and the necessary corrections, but you must develop an ability to assess by inner perception. Competent postural correction requires an awareness of your own body, followed by a quick adjustment of position.

11. Posture in standing

Basic principles

The best way of giving advice on postural correction is through one-to-one communication – a book can only communicate basic principles. Many books merely advise 'standing tall' or offer other imprecise instructions. Postural correction is covered here in as much detail as possible, and taken step by step. When you have decided which postural type you are, you might ask someone else to read out the instructions while you alter the pose; it should then be easier to follow the necessary steps to reach a new, correct stance.

Precise postural rules are open to dispute as naturally inherited familial and racial characteristics must be taken into account. Certain families and races have a greater lordosis while others have a flatter back; in such cases correction might be unwarranted. All physical disability is unique to the individual, and the adjustments described here might not be applicable.

Perfect posture should ideally be a position of easy balance, a balance of bone on bone. It should require a minimum of effort to maintain but provide maximum mobility and function. Because perfect posture should contain no tension, any postural correction which demands excessive, awkward muscular tightening has to be incorrect and is unsustainable.

Postural correction must never be an awkward pulling or pushing or forcing of parts of the body into a new shape. It is a re-positioning, not of one isolated section but of one part on the other, gently, all the way up from the feet to the head, a realignment of the body as a whole. For example, the most misguided advice ever given to amend 'round shoulders' is to 'Pull your shoulders back!' – an exhortation often heard from drill sergeants and well-meaning parents alike.

It is important to understand the reasons why this frequent correction is of no value. The **shoulder girdle**, the whole mobile area connected to the shoulder tips, consists of the **clavicle** (collarbone) in front and the **scapula** (shoulder blade) at the back. These meet to form a roof over the top of the **humerus** (upper arm), while the side of the scapula provides the **glenoid cavity** for articulation with the humerus, thus forming the **shoulder joint**. The whole structure is joined to the skeleton at only one bony point, where the clavicle meets the **sternum** (breastbone) in front;

otherwise the connections are purely muscular. Pulling the shoulders back therefore has no influence at all on the spinal curves.

For this reason the shoulders have been omitted intentionally from all illustrations. In **11.1**, if the imaginary shoulders were pulled back at their tips there would no change of position of the spine, merely a tendency to thrust the chin further forwards, creating increased tension in the area. In perfect posture, while the spine is held in correct alignment, the shoulders should be allowed to drop, not droop, into comfortable relaxation – without allowing the chest to cave in.

Common postural deviations

The three most common deviations from perfect posture are shown in **11.1**, I shall refer to them as the **flat back**, the **hollow back** and the **sway back**.

11.1

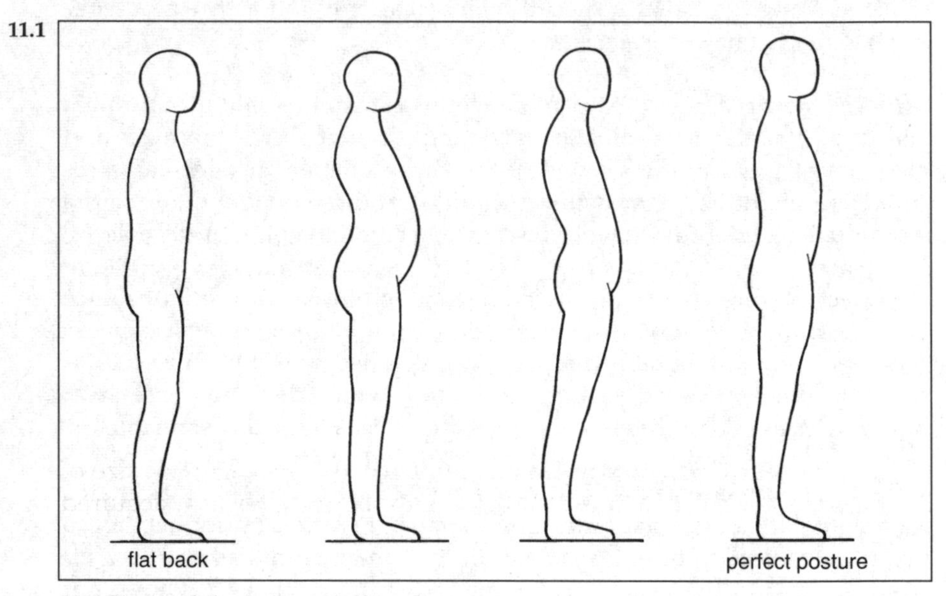

11.1 Postural deviations and good posture

Each postural type must first be considered in an overall appraisal, surveying the entire bodily alignment centred around an imaginary plumb line dropped to the ground from just behind the ear. The line should fall through the centre of the shoulder joint, through the centre of the hip joint, towards the front of the knee, to end up just in front of the ankles. This gives the body a slightly forwards inclination, the weight more towards the ball of the foot than the heels (**11.2**).

Perfect posture

In perfect standing the chest is the farthest point forwards, the buttocks the farthest point backwards and the body is aligned evenly around the

11.2

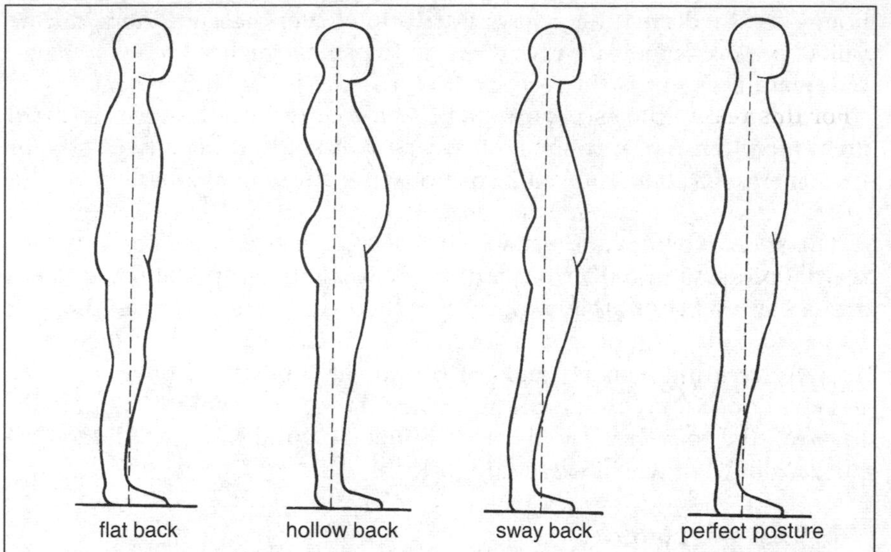

11.2 Deviations from the centre of gravity (plumb line dropped from behind the ears)

plumb line. This position allows the skeletal components, bone on bone, to balance in a way that requires merely the gentlest muscle tone to hold it there, maintaining the three vertebral curves in their ideal, natural position. The opposing muscle groups will be interacting with each other in an effortless, balanced way without having to grapple with awkward local corrections or, conversely, without being allowed to slacken and lengthen to the point of relinquishing all joint support.

The flat back

The flat back often results from an attempt to conceal the apparent size of the buttocks and breasts; it is also the elderly person's hazard, acquired through too many hours spent sitting and stooping, unaware of the need to restore the lordosis, the loss of which is the obvious fault of this posture. However, correction of the lordosis without looking further would neglect a fundamental point – in this posture the knees are invariably held in flexion. Omission of this point would add stress to the overall remodelling.

The hollow back and sway back

The hollow back and the sway back have a certain similarity which makes them more difficult to diagnose, sometimes causing confusion over postural correction. The similarity lies in the lordosis. Both postures have an increased lordosis but each stems from a different, almost opposite, source and therefore requires a quite different correction.

The **hollow back lordosis** has the hips flexed; the buttocks are thrust well back; the knees vary, they can be bent or pressed back; the abdomen hangs forward creating a huge lordotic curve; the shoulders can be pulled back or rounded with a thoracic kyphosis; the head tends to hang; the overall weight is thrust back towards the heels. This resembles an uncorrected toddler's posture which never quite attained the right abdominal tension to solve the forward pelvic tilt; it usually originates from increased abdominal bulk and/or weak abdominal muscle.

The **sway back lordosis** is a result of allowing the hips to sway forwards, pressing into the front of the over-extended hip joints; the knees are usually pressed back hard; the chest collapses inwards; the thoracic spine sways back in order to compensate for the pelvic swing forwards, actually creating a sharp angle at the lower lumbar spine; finally, the neck scoops to create a poking chin. The overall weight is usually towards the toes. It is the most common postural fault, the hands-in-pocket slouch of which we are all guilty.

In these two postures:

- The shape of the lordotic increase is different: the sway back being a sharp angle in the lower lumbar spine, the hollow back being an enlarged wide sweep from buttocks to thoracic spine.
- The body alignment which originated the increase stems from an almost opposing alteration in skeletal balance.

If the two postures are corrected in the same manner, by alteration of pelvic tilt, the sway back will be heading for an untenable posture, possibly with increased trouble rather than relief.

Deviations from the ideal posture start from different points, for many different reasons. So in postural correction, it is essential to find the lowest point at fault, even if it is not the most obvious, and correct that first. Then, the final correction must be the adjustment of the centre of gravity so that it falls through the body in the right way, ending towards the front of the ankles.

To get a clear feeling for this, stand sideways on to a long mirror and look at your own posture. Can you decide which postural type you are? Now do a few alterations to your body to see what happens. Press your knees back and then slacken them several times slowly, watching your back; note how the movement affects the angle of your pelvis.

Now slacken your knees, pull in your abdomen, flattening the lumbar spine, and let your chest drop slightly – you should be in a flat back position. Change now to: knees pressed back, buttocks stuck out backwards, abdomen projecting forwards and shoulders pulled back – have you found the hollow back? Now put your hands in your pockets if you have them, let your hips sway forwards with your knees pressed back, let your chest collapse and your top body sway back behind your hips –

a bit like the catwalk model's posture; you should be looking like the sway back.

Here's another experiment. Stand with your weight really far back on your heels. Can you feel what is happening to your toes? Are they tending to curl up and lift from the ground? Now transfer your weight slowly towards the balls of your feet – you should feel your toes spreading out and tending to flatten on the ground. Posture also affects toe movement and toe health. A posture maintained with weight permanently on the heels will eventually have a deleterious effect upon the toes.

Feet play a vital role in the growing structural development of the body. They are the base on which the skeletal structures stand; any deformity or inaccuracy of this base can effect the whole edifice, altering the knees, the hips and finally the back. **Podiatry**, the study and treatment of foot irregularities, specialises in careful examination of the feet. Podiatrists and physiotherapists take video films of the body in action to search out problems, using slow-motion shots to analyse the components of movement and the measurement of various angles of alignment. If 'flat feet' or other foot irregularities were rectified early in life many postural defects could be avoided.

Postural correction in standing

General rules for maintaining postural correction

In each postural deviation there is usually one crucial fault that includes a lengthening and weakening of a particular muscle group. Comerford (1993) suggests that correction of this should become a 'red-dot' exercise; he suggests that you should stick little red-dot stickers all over the house or work place and every time you see one you do your postural correction or special postural 'hold'. While maintaining this correction or hold, try not to become rigid all over, relax your head, shoulders and body without letting any part sag again, and move around normally, continuing with work. Achieving and maintaining this 'hold' will become easier as you get to know your body, as you begin to *feel* the difference in positioning and as your muscles start to respond to the gentle movement.

At the end of each postural correction there will be advice about corrective exercises and a suggestion for the 'red-dot' hold. Because postural correction is such a personal need, the 'red-dot' might not, in fact, be exactly right for you – so, if it does not feel right, or if it causes or increases pain, do not continue with it. In all diagrams of this section, where one posture is superimposed on another, the faulty posture is drawn in continuous line with perfect posture in dotted line.

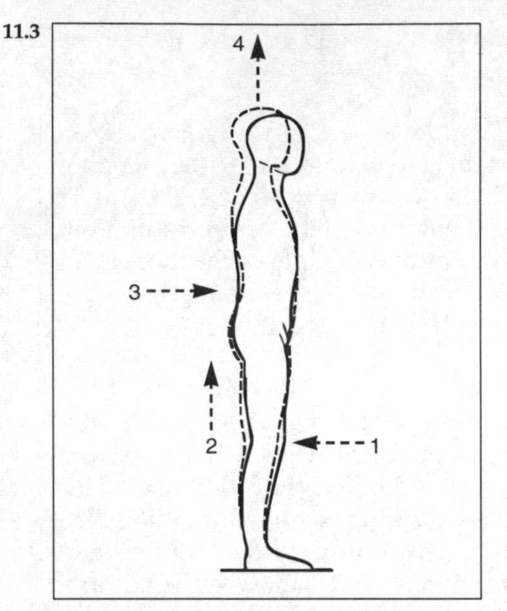

11.3 Postural correction for the flat back

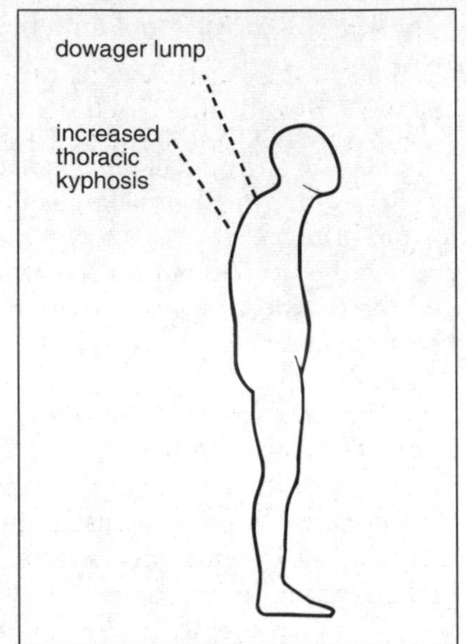

11.4 The ageing flat back

Flat back

Salient points: flexed knees, flattened lumbar spine, loss of all curves, chest dropped.

Aims of correction: to increase the lordosis; raise and open the chest (**11.3**):

1 Start by straightening the knees. This will help towards attaining (2) + (3)
2 Tip the pelvis forwards a little, raising the buttocks.
3 Increase the lordotic arch with a gentle stretch of the chest, pushing it forwards and up, arching the thoracic spine. Keep the shoulders relaxed, but do not drop your chest as you relax your shoulders. Check that the overall weight is mid-foot.
4 Add a feeling of growing tall.

Exercises: Having achieved this posture, if your back is pain-free a gentle regime of exercises is necessary. Exercises should mobilise the lumbar spine, strengthen the back extensor muscles, strengthen the hip extensor and quadriceps muscles, stretch the front of the hips.

Red-dot: Gently arch the back to increase the lordosis.

If the flat back is not corrected, **11.4** can develop. There is the same flat lumbar spine but an additional increased thoracic kyphosis and dowager hump. Correction is as above but the accent should be on mobilising and exercising the thoracic spine with chin retraction exercises for the neck. (See Chapter 18, p. 197 and 205). If this is happening to you, start now to work to correct it. Remember, this is the danger area for osteoporosis and exercise is the best remedy.

The hollow back

Salient points: knees can be pressed back or flexed; increased forward pelvic tilt with the buttocks projecting backwards; hips flexed; shoulders pulled back; weight on the heels.

Aims of correction: to decrease the lordosis, stretch the hips, strengthen the abdominal muscles. In this example the knees are presumed to be pressed back (**11.5**):

1 Slacken the knees. This allows the buttocks to drop a little.
2 Gently tighten the abdominal muscles and the buttock muscles to tip the pelvis back, decreasing the lordosis.
3 Shift the chest forwards, not back. This helps to smooth out the lordosis from the top and also brings the centre of gravity forwards to mid-foot.
4 Add a feeling of growing tall.

11.5

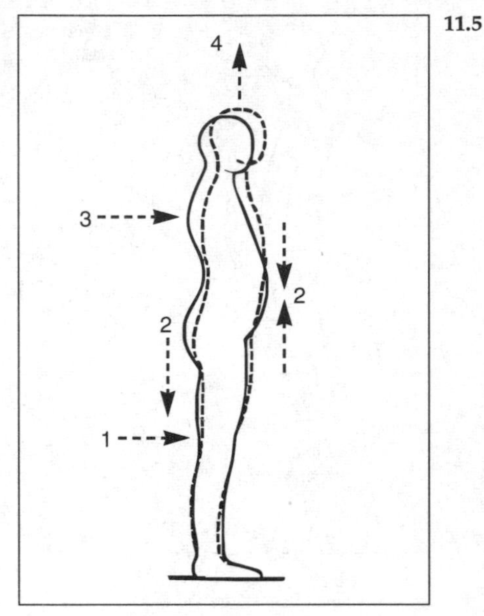

11.5 Postural correction for the hollow back

Exercises: If pain-free, the following exercises are necessary: abdominal exercises; exercises for mobilising and flexing the lumbar spine; hip extensor exercises; hip flexor stretching (stretching the joint into extension). Flexion postures for pain relief may be necessary after any prolonged standing (see **9.3** p. 115).

Red-dot: abdominal hollowing (p. 201) and gentle buttock tightening.

The sway back

The moves in this postural correction may be difficult to accomplish because of the several unfamiliar shifts of direction, but once achieved it is surprisingly easy to become adept at instantaneous correction.

Salient points: hips thrust forwards; knees pressed back; chest dropped with resulting rounding of the thoracic spine; upper body slumped backwards; poking chin; weight towards the front of the feet.

11.6 compares the sway back with perfect posture and may help to clarify the faults.

11.6

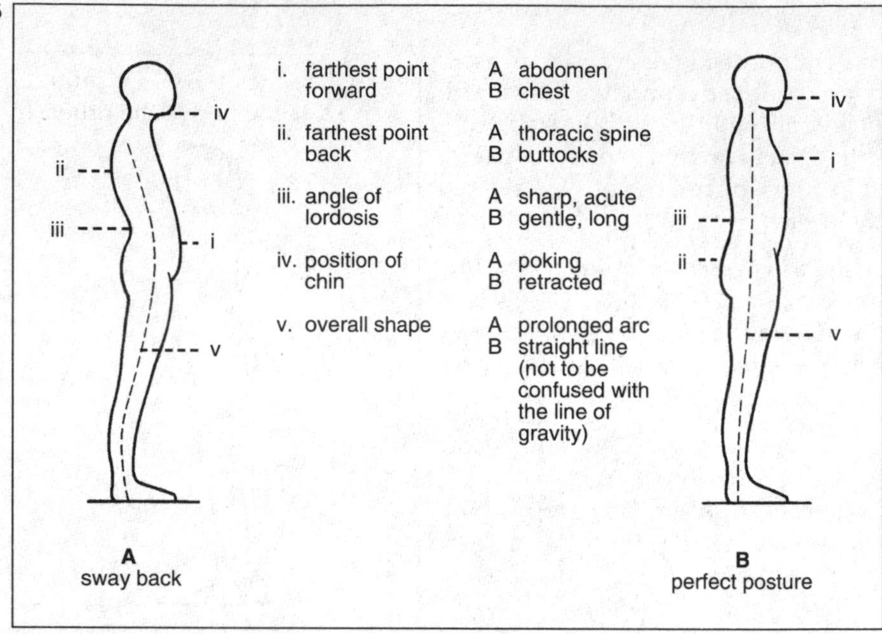

11.6 Comparing the sway back with perfect posture

Aims of correction: to think in terms of body 'realignment', adjusting one part on the other. It is most important to remain relaxed and to feel this movement rather than force it (**11.7**).

1 Transfer the whole body weight back onto the heels with an easy backward sway of the hips. Do not tighten the abdominal muscles or tip the pelvis intentionally.
2 Keeping the body steady from the waist down, shift the chest forwards at the point of the sternum (breastbone) as if someone were poking a gun between the shoulder blades. Do not arch back. Do not pull the shoulders back. The shoulders should be relaxed but beware! – do not collapse the chest as the shoulders relax.
3 Retract the chin, stretching the back of the head as if hanging from the ceiling like a puppet with a rope right down through the spine.

11.7

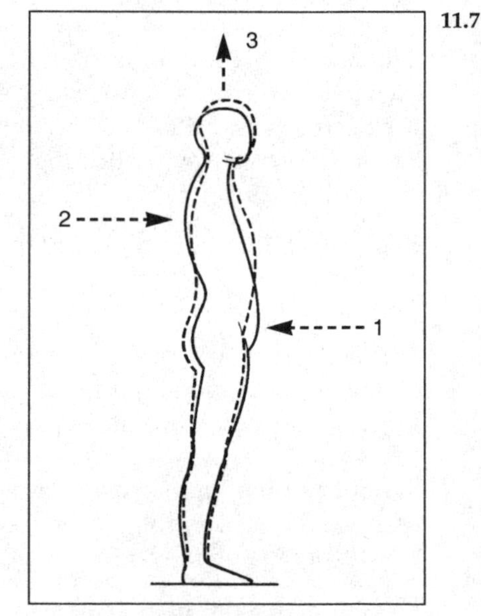

11.7 Postural correction for the sway back

Other ways of thinking: after correcting (1) in **11.7**, imagine you are standing facing a chest-high fence; raise the chest forwards and up to look over the fence while leaving the hips where they were. Or think of the two areas of the body as two boxes as in **11.8**, one above the other. In the sway back the lower box has shifted forwards and the upper one has glided backwards. To correct, they must be pushed in the opposite direction. In this correction there should be no tension. Every alteration should be a gentle repositioning rather than a forced hold.

11.8

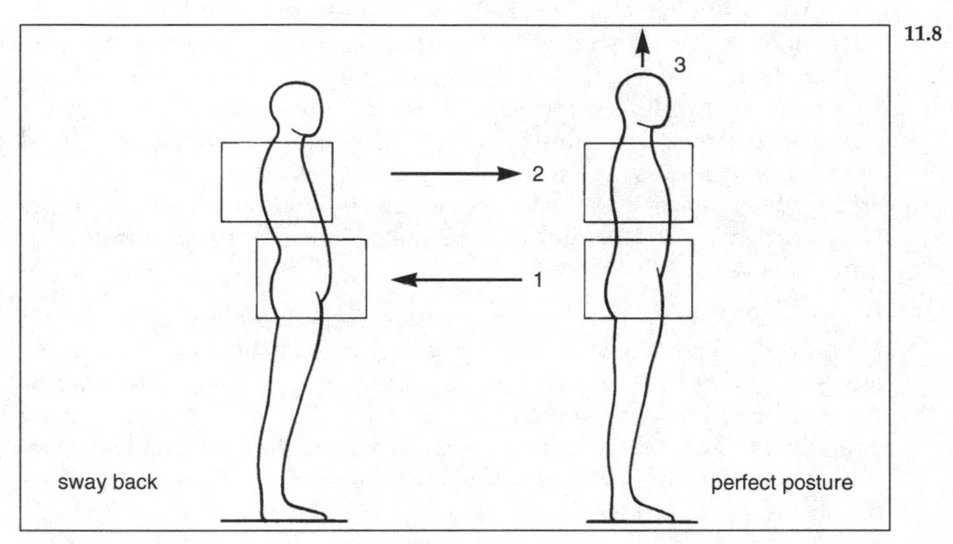

11.8 Diagrammatic example of sway back correction

Exercises: If pain-free the following exercises are necessary: all exercises for thoracic extension, especially exercises 18.7-9 p. 197-198; abdominal muscles exercises; poking chin correction; general mobilising exercises for the lumbar spine and hips.

Red-dot: exercise number 18.9, performed without the table; constant postural correction.

Care in standing

Having corrected your standing posture, the next step in back care is to avoid long periods of standing. No doubt all those people in standing jobs will give a hollow laugh. However, if you follow the rules below maybe you can keep your job, stay pain-free, and feel you have a life to live after work.

- Never slouch or prop yourself against the nearest upright; leaning around is guaranteed to end in exhaustion.
- Keep a wide base in standing, feet slightly apart, even standing with one leg slightly in front of the other but...

- Always keep your weight evenly distributed between both feet and your relaxed, corrected posture maintained.
- Keep your knees relaxed in a comfortably straight position, avoid pressing them back more and more as time passes but likewise avoid letting them bend.
- Rest one foot up on a low stool or step (if available), for short periods. This changes the position of your lumbar spine and can give relief.
- Move around as much as you can, if only to shift position.
- Move the lumbar spine. Every 10–15 minutes put your hands into the small of the back and arch backwards (see **9.1** p. 113). If you have an increased lordosis, rock your pelvis forwards and back or bend forwards into flexion for a few seconds. Movement of the lumbar spine in either direction or in both directions increases the local circulation, moves the tissues and reduces pain.
- Your feet, especially your toes, must be able to function freely. If toes are curled up and painful in your shoes, postural balance cannot be maintained.

High heels affect posture in different ways depending upon the particular postural type. However, their effect is largely dependent upon the ankle mobility of the wearer. Loose, supple, ballerina-type ankles allow the foot in high heels to be comfortably pointed while the knees remain straight and the lumbar lordosis unaffected, though there might be a tendency towards an increased lordosis. However, with restricted ankle point, the angle at the ankle is limited, the knees remain pulled forwards, and the body tends to tip forwards with flexed knees and a flattened lordosis. Unless you are especially used to them, try to avoid wearing high heels for long periods, especially for tiring events like shopping and sightseeing.

Flat shoes are preferable to high heels as they leave the foot less restricted, providing the toes are not of the excessively pointed variety; they allow for better heel-toe action in walking and they interfere less with the foot/body postural relationship. However, if you have shortened calf muscles and find that flat shoes give a pain at the back of your legs, then you should wear slightly raised heels, or try to stretch your calf muscles by daily exercises to enable you to wear flat shoes with comfort.

Foot posture does affect the back and so it is worth studying the relationship between your shoes, your legs and your posture to avoid any stress that may originate in this way.

REFERENCES

Comerford, M. (1993) (personal communication).

12. *Posture in sitting*

Basic principles

We spend hours sitting every day – but rarely in a good position. There are two reasons for this: one is our lack of awareness, the other is that our misdemeanour is encouraged by appalling chair design. Now that you have read Part 1, the first of these excuses should be invalid – and now that ergonomic advice is easily available to manufacturers, the second excuse should soon be inapplicable.

The escalating frequency of back, neck and arm problems in office workers in recent years has led to increased scientific examination of body mechanics in the sitting posture.

In sitting, the pelvis rotates backwards and the lumbar spine tends to fall into flexion, accumulating all the stresses generated by sustained flexion. The lumbar intervertebral discs are compressed anteriorly and stretched posteriorly with greatly increased intradiscal pressure (see **3.5,** p. 36).

Research into intradiscal pressure in the sitting posture has shown that pressure in sitting is least in the supported, upright or slightly inclined backwards posture, but it increases with removal of the support and increases yet further when leaning forwards with a flexed lumbar spine (Andersson *et al.*, 1975, Andersson *et al* ., 1979).

The position of the knees is crucial to the degree of curve in the lumbar spine (Keegan, 1953). The higher the knees are raised, the greater the curve (**12.1**). This is relevant to the angle of inclination of chair seats: the further the seat is tipped backwards, the higher the knees are raised in front and the more the lumbar spine is forced into flexion.

12.1

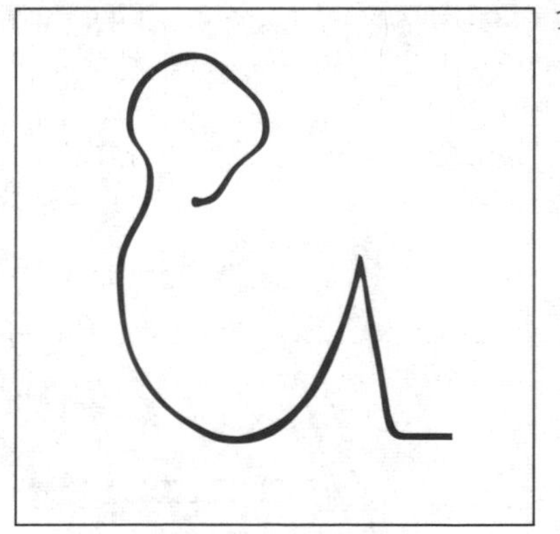

12.1 Sitting with knees high

12.2

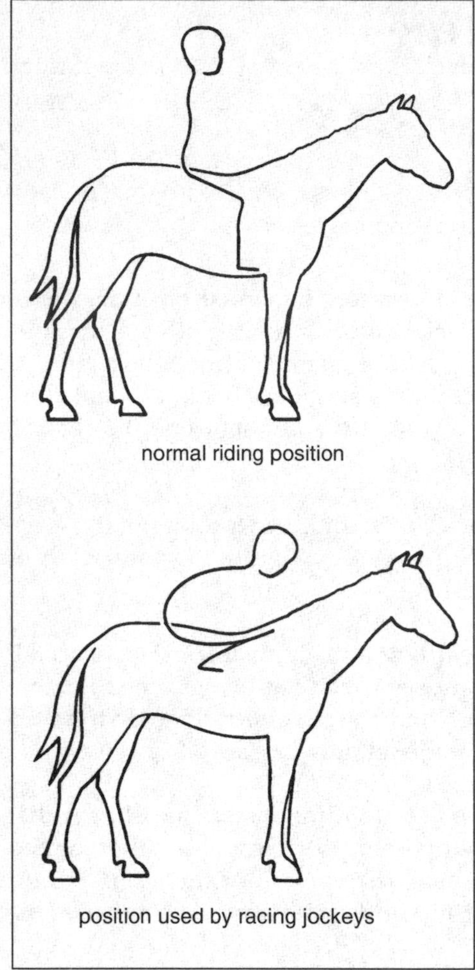

12.2 The effect of change of leg position on the lumbar spine

The lower the thighs are placed, the easier it is to maintain the lumbar lordosis. The optimum comfort of the lumbar spine is achieved when the legs are placed at about 45° of hip flexion (Keegan, 1953). A forward sloping seat would mimic this position.

A good example of the influence of leg position upon the lumbar spine can be seen when comparing a normal riding position with the position used by the modern racing jockey (**12.2**). In the former the legs are supported in stirrups in the position of 45° hip flexion and the lumbar lordosis is well maintained; in the latter the shortened stirrups bring the hips and knees into almost complete flexion forcing the lumbar spine into an excessive curve.

The comfort of the sloping thigh position has been used by generations of children who spontaneously tip their chairs forwards when working at a desk or table (Mandall, 1984). The principle was adopted by the Balans chair, designed and manufactured in Norway (**12.3**), and is now being incorporated into the design of all office chairs which offer a wide choice of seat adaptability.

12.3

12.3 Balans chair – basic design

General chair design

The ideal chair should be one in which the hips can be placed right at the back of the seat whilst the thighs are well supported, with no upward pressure against the thighs and no pressure behind the knees. Both feet should rest easily on the floor. There should be good support in the back rest, especially in the lumbar area, maintaining the lordosis and preventing a slump into flexion. The chair should be easy to sit in and rise from without effort or struggle.

Every chair should be a source of support, not of abuse. It should contribute, both at work and at leisure, to the efficiency and comfort of life at all times by:

- Reducing physical strain and fatigue in any sedentary job.
- Providing a restorative day-time break for physically active workers, such as a comfortable bar stool, (possibly of the Balans design) or good dining chair – thus avoiding one of the risk situations of slouching when physically tired.
- Supplying unstressed relaxation at the end of a day in a public or private place. Theatre and cinema seats are notoriously provocative, possibly because of their tipped-back inclination.

The basic principle is that sitting as in (**12.4**) is to be avoided and sitting as in (**12.5**) is correct.

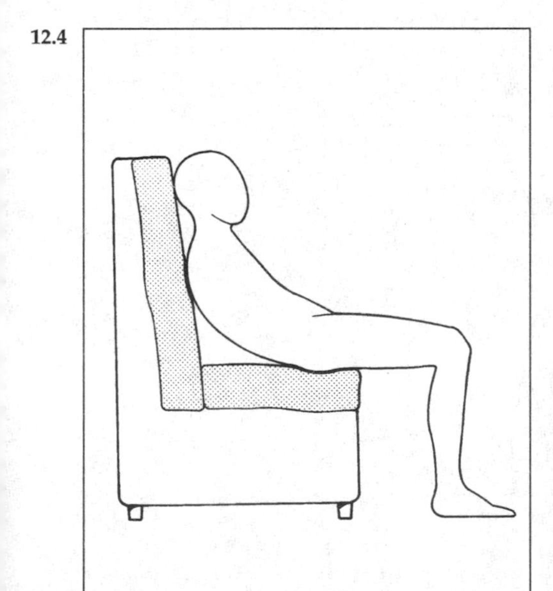

12.4 Sitting – the wrong way

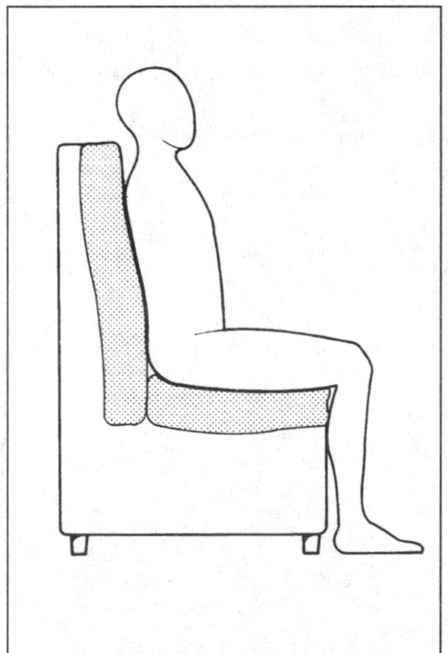

12.5 Sitting – the right way

This principle applies to all backs at all times, apart from certain high lumbar lesions and conditions of spondylolisthesis which are more comfortable sitting in slight lumbar flexion, well supported nevertheless.

The office chair

Chair design should never be considered in isolation but always as an integral part of task and workshop design (Brunswick, 1984).

The seat

- The length of the seat should be less than the length of the thighs.
- The seat should be rounded on the front edge to avoid upward pressure
- The seat angle should be adjustable to facilitate variation in the slope from front to back. The angle of inclination should be adaptable from 5–15° (Mandall, 1984). If you work from home, using an ordinary chair, it is possible to buy wedges which create the downward slope and can be used in any chair (**12.6**). Be careful not to buy a wedge that is too steep. However, in those few clinical conditions mentioned previously where the spine is more comfortable in slight flexion the seat needs to be adjusted the other way, slightly raising the knees by 5°.
- The seat should be upholstered in non-slip, comfortable material.

Height from the floor

- The height from the floor should be such that both feet can rest on the floor whilst the seat supports the thighs without upward pressure. Office chairs should have a height adjustment facility to accommodate changes in worktop levels.
- Foot rests should be used if the seat is too high and cannot be altered.

12.6

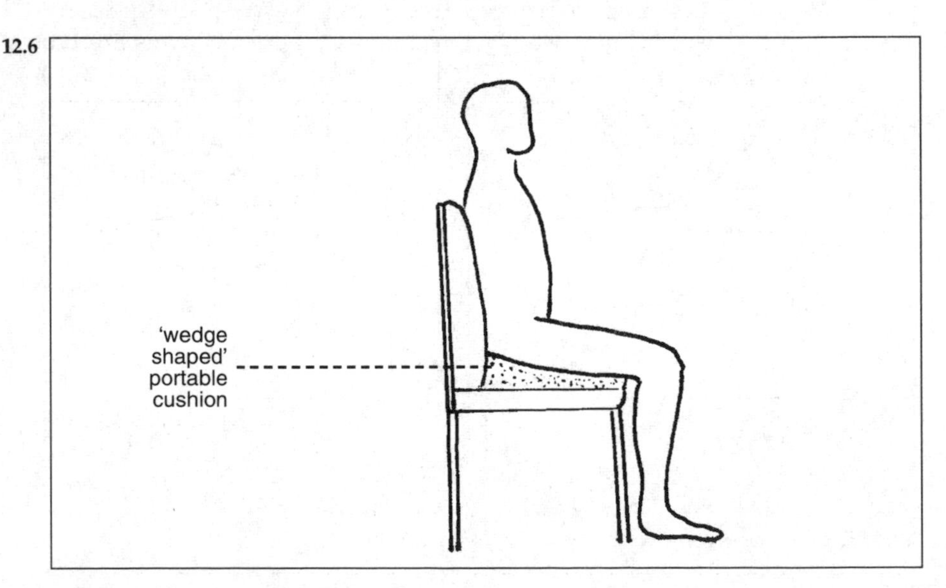

12.6 Portable seat inclination cushion

The back rest

- The back rest should be firm but not hard, with a convex curve to provide lumbar support at waist level.
- The height and inclination of the back rest should be adjustable. The correct inclination depends upon the position of the head and the angle of work in relation to the eyes. The angle should be adjustable between 90 and 100° (Boyling, 1992), though some visual display unit (VDU) operators have chosen inclinations varying from 104–110°, depending upon the position of their screens (Hayne, 1984) (see the section on VDU operators, p. 162).

The width of the chair

The width of the chair should be sufficient to accommodate both hips comfortably and allow easy change of position.

The base of the chair

- Office chairs should be on a five-star, swivel base to allow for quick change of direction without awkward movement. The base should be wider than the seat for stability.
- All chairs should be on good castors for easy moving (see **12.7**).

Lever adjustments

All lever adjustments should be comfortable to use and easy to operate.

Armrests in all chairs

Armrests should be high enough to support the arms with elbows bent at a right angle, avoiding upward pressure on the elbow. Knitters and needleworkers should be careful to avoid using chairs where the armrests get in the way of their elbow movement; if the chair arms are too

12.7

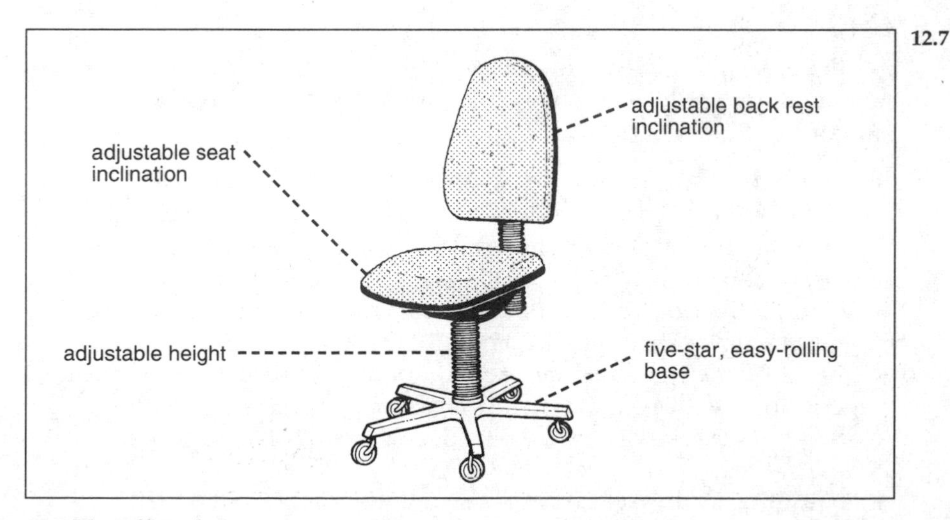

12.7 The office chair

high or if the chair is too narrow, the lack of freedom will encourage hunched shoulders and tension in the neck and shoulder area.

The easy chair

All the rules of lumbar and leg support apply equally to easy chairs and considering the amount of time we spend in them, a good chair is of paramount importance.

- In view of the paucity of good design, careful consideration should be given to the depth of the seat before you purchase any new chair. A common fault, made in the name of 'luxury', is a depth so exaggerated that the average person is quite unable to sit right back in the chair with both feet remaining on the floor, see **12.4**. and **12.5**.
- The chair should provide good lumbar support to preserve the lordosis while you relax in a non-stressful position.
- The chair should be large enough to allow easy change of position yet small enough to give support where necessary.
- The back inclination of an easy chair should not be less than 105° but if it is greater than 120° there should be adequate head support (Liston 1987).

Rocking chairs

Use of the rocking chair is strongly recommended by Wyke (1987) as a therapeutic means of reducing pain. The rhythmical oscillations of the body as it rocks to and fro generate soothing discharges from the mechanoreceptors located in the moving joints and muscles. These maintain a prolonged inhibitory blockade of the painful input – an example of the gate control mechanism working in everyday life. The rocking chair also assists pulmonary ventilation and augments the venous return from the lower limbs (ibid).

Car seats

All these design guidelines apply to car seats. Some manufacturers are now designing fully-adaptable seats with individually-adjustable lumbar supports in the back rest.

- Adjust the seat carefully to arrive at the best degree of support all round. Driving is a stressful activity, causing postural awkwardness in wheel turning and gear changing, to say nothing of the emotional tension of motorway madness (Twomey and Taylor 1987).
- Sit at the right distance from the pedals to enable easy, unstrained leg movement. Keep the hips well into the back of the seat.
- The seat back should be inclined at about 105° so that driving can be performed with bent arms. Leaning back and steering with straight arms puts excessive strain upon the thoracic spine, especially at the base of the neck.
- Adjust the headrest close to the back of the head (**12.8**).

12.8

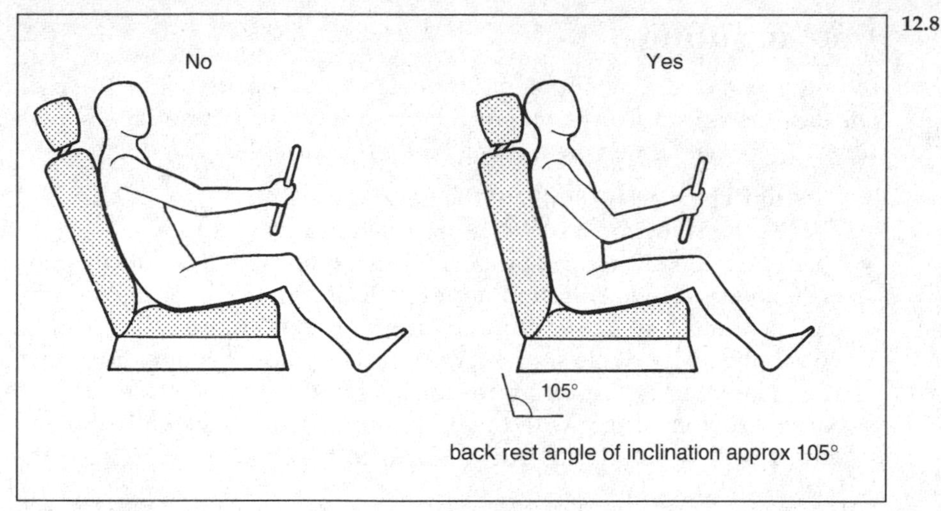

12.8 Car seats

Casual chairs

If a particular lifestyle entails frequent changes of environment with different chairs, some lacking adequate lumbar support, it is advisable to take a small cushion around, moving it from chair to chair when necessary. There are several different lumbar support cushions or rolls on the market but it is advisable to try to borrow one on approval first to test it thoroughly before buying (**12.9**).

12.9

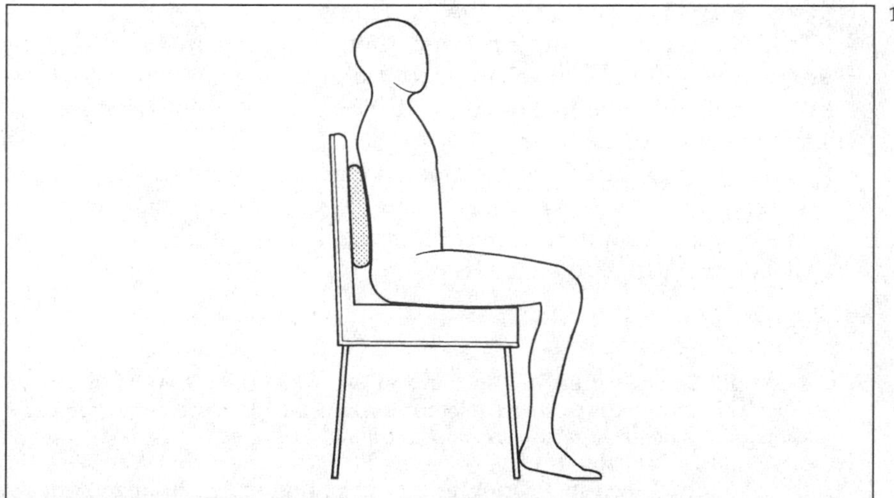

12.9 Portable lumbar support cushion

Care in sitting

Sitting is one of the most potentially provocative positions for the back and for this reason it is essential to be aware of our sitting habits at all times. There is no time when sitting badly is excusable.

- Hips must be placed right into the back of the seat.
- The lumbar spine must be well supported in a good lordosis.
- Do not remain sitting in one position for long periods, shift position or stand up and walk around at intervals. Every 15–20 minutes slump the back into a relaxed rounded position, then arch it. This can be done quite easily while sitting. When driving, stop, get out and stretch at regular intervals, restoring the lordosis with an arch back.
- Never rise from sitting with the back rounded and then walk off to do things with it remaining in the slumped position. Always arch the back as in **9.1**, p. 113.
- Do not sit with both legs up on a stool unless this is necessary for other medical reasons; the position pulls the lumbar spine into flexion and applies stress to the back. If poor lower limb circulation or any other condition does require this position, then, instead of sitting up straight, allow the back to recline at a greater angle while adding plenty of lumbar support.
- Avoid crossing the legs at the knees, it exerts a twisting strain on the back – and it is bad for veins!
- Do not sit for hours on the floor propped against furniture with both legs straight out in front – this also pulls the lumbar spine into flexion and applies stress to the back. If this position is being used in exercise class or other therapy that is a different matter; the difference is between a long sustained position that strains and a short stretch that can be beneficial. If the floor is your favourite spot for sitting, then change poses frequently. Use cushions for extra support.
- Get into a car by sitting first and then swinging in your legs. Be especially careful if you are in a painful or 'twingeing' episode. Care at moments like this makes all the difference between irritating and protecting a potential injury.
- Beware of sitting up in bed, propped on numerous pillows, reading or watching television – especially if you have back pain. Provide ample lumbar support. Shift position frequently. Always move and arch the back before settling down to sleep.

REFERENCES

Andersson, B.J.G., Ortengren, R., Nachemson, A.L., Elstrom, G.,and Broman, H. (1975). The sitting posture. An electromyographic and discometric study, *Orthopaedic Clinics of North America* **6**(1), 105–120.

Andersson, B.J.G., Murphy, R.W., Ortengren, R., and Nachemson, A. (1979). The influence of back rest inclination and lumbar support on lumbar lordosis, *Spine*, **4**(1), 52–58.

Boyling, J.D. (1992). (personal communication).
Brunswick, M. (1984). Ergonomics of seat design, *Physiotherapy*, **70**(2).
Hayne, C. R. (1984). Ergonomics and back pain, *Physiotherapy*, **70**(1).
Keegan, J.J. (1953). Alterations of the lumbar curve related to posture and seating, *J. Bone Joint Surg.*, **35**, 589–603.
Liston, C.B. (1987). Back school and ergonomics, *Physical Therapy of the Low Back* (Twomey, L.T. and Taylor, J.R., eds.), Churchill Livingstone.
Mandall, A.C. (1984). The correct height of school furniture, *Physiotherapy*, **70**(2).
Twomey, L.T. and Taylor, J.R. (1987). The lumbar spine, low back pain, and physical therapy, *Physical Therapy of the Low Back*, (Twomey, L.T. and Taylor, J.R., eds.), Churchill Livingstone.
Wyke, B. (1987). The neurology of low back pain, *The Lumbar Spine and Back Pain* (Jayson, M.I.V., ed.), 3rd ed., Churchill Livingstone.

13. Posture in lying

Basic principles

There are no rules about the way in which you should lie. Lie in the most comfortable position for you. Allow yourself to move and spread around the bed as much as you need. Enjoy stretching out your body in this relaxed situation.

When in pain, follow the advice suggested in 'coping with an acute attack' on p. 181. Ignore all gratuitous advice about positions you 'ought' to use, and lie in any position that provides relief and enables you to sleep. Sleep is indispensable in the healing process.

However, what you sleep *on* is important.

Bed design

Medical opinion used to be in favour of extra-firm beds, even to the extent of advocating sleeping on the floor. Gradually we have come to realise that the body contours are unsupported on a hard surface, with gravity tending to influence the direction of the spinal curves; if these curves are without buttress during sleep they are under stress.

Hard beds

The effects on the spine when sleeping on a hard surface are shown in **13.1** and **13.2**. Lying supine (**13.1**) the lumbar spine is either unsupported as in the diagram or it falls into flexion with the pull of gravity flattening the curve. In side lying, the waist is unsupported, so the lumbar spine falls into a scoliotic-type curve towards the mattress (**13.2**).

Soft beds

Soft beds are the worst of all evils; they sag in the middle where the body is heaviest encouraging loss of good spinal shape in every position (**13.3, 13.4**).

Firm beds

The ideal bed has a very firm base with a mattress that is sensitive to small changes of pressure on the surface, accommodating superficially to all the body protuberances but remaining supportive of natural body hollows. It undulates on the surface but remains firm in the depths (**13.5, 13.6**).

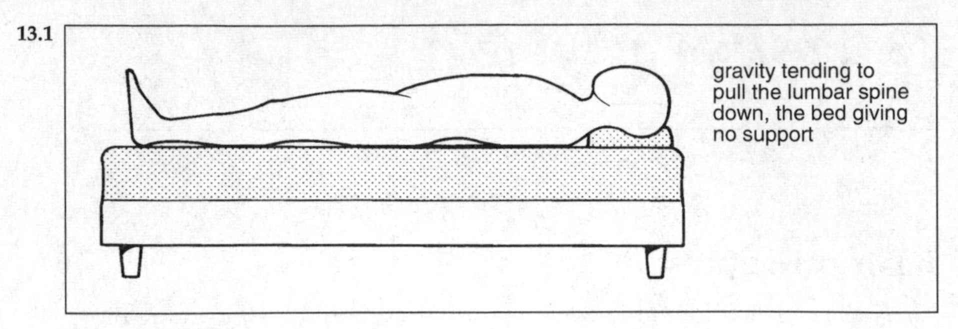

13.1 A hard bed

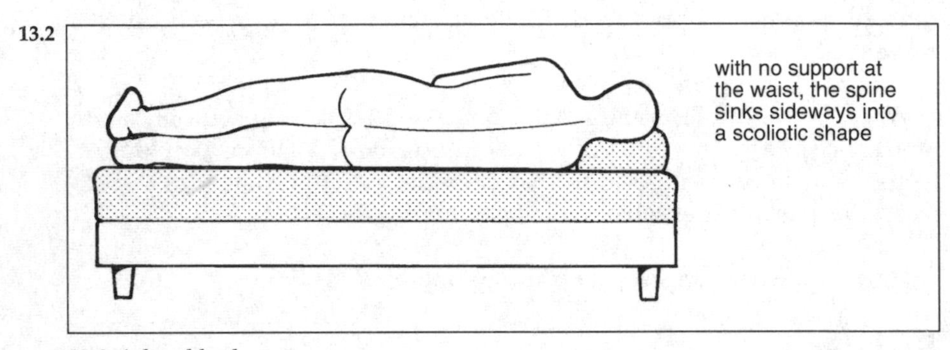

13.2 A hard bed

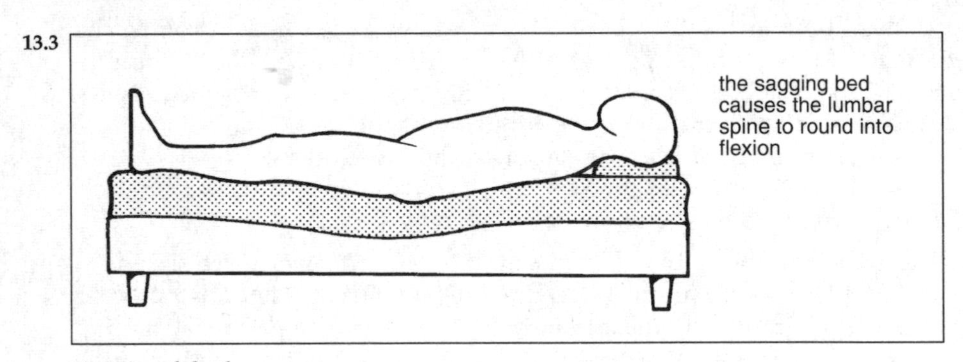

13.3 A soft bed

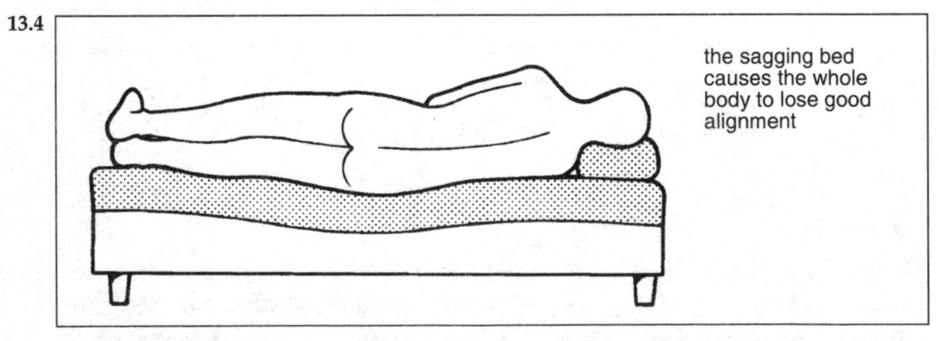

13.4 A soft bed

13.5

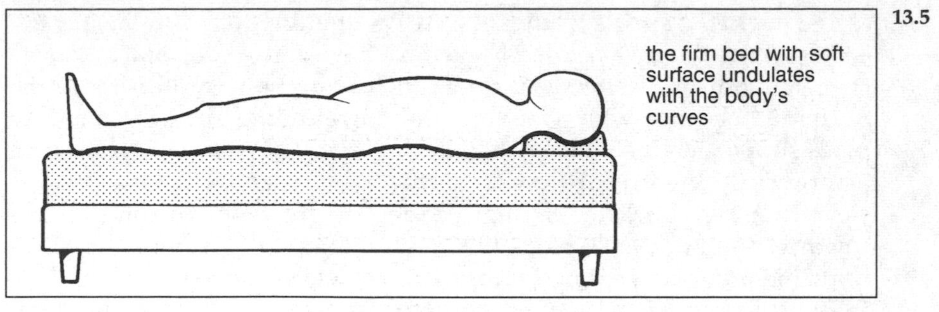

13.5 A firm bed

13.6

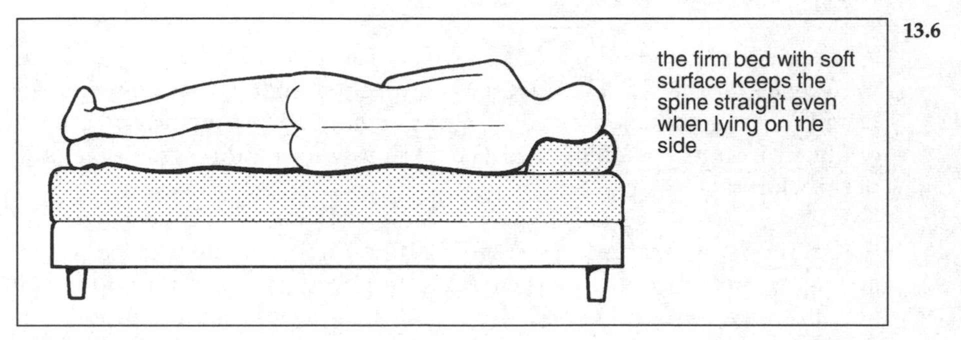

13.6 A firm bed

Mattress construction

Mattresses can be made from springs, from foam or latex, or they can be water-filled. Sprung mattresses are constructed in three different ways: the open coil, the continuous coil and the pocketed spring (*Which?* 1991). Some manufacturers combine one or more methods.

The **open coil** springing system, which is the most commonly-used type, consists of rows of hour-glass shaped upright springs joined together along the top and the bottom by a continuous small diameter spiral spring (NBF, 1988). The perimeter of the mattress is strengthened by the use of a heavy gauge border rod both at the top and bottom of the mattress (ibid). Movement is linked all the way through the line of springs so that an indentation at one point has a knock-on effect over a large area. The firmness depends upon two criteria: the number of springs used and the tension of the slings. If these slings are taut, the mattress is extremely firm, scarcely giving at all, but if they slacken with wear, the mattress can sag like a hammock.

The **continuous open coil** is made by forming a single length of wire into coils up and down the mattress. The result is the softest and possibly the most luxurious feel, but with minimal support.

The **pocketed spring** mattress has rows of individual upright springs, each surrounded by a padded pocket, each working independently from its neighbour (NBF, 1988). At the point of any bony protuberance the individual springs will give while the surrounding springs remain in place supporting the hollows. In this way every part of the body is constantly supported regardless of positional change. When two people sleep in a bed, pocketed springs reduce the tendency to roll together towards the middle (*Which?* 1991). The degree of firmness depends upon the number of springs in the mattress, which can be from 500–1200 (NBF, 1988), so a pocketed spring mattress can vary from being relatively soft to extremely firm.

A variety of different materials are used for the top padding, and the preference for one kind or another is entirely a matter of personal taste. Details of types of bases, padding and general bed-buying advice can be obtained from the National Bed Federation whose address is at the end of this chapter.

'**Orthopaedic**' mattresses often combine the open coil and pocketed spring, achieving the firmest possible support; but the label does not actually mean anything, and they have no special medical properties (NBF, 1988). If you have one of these beds and you are happy with it, keep it. However, if you are about to purchase a new bed, ignore all publicity and be careful to choose one that gives adequate support but one which suits you, not one that you feel you 'ought' to have.

Foam and **latex** mattresses have improved in construction in recent years; the variation of firmness can now be adjusted in a similar way to sprung systems in order to provide different degrees of support, often constructed with a firmer layer at the bottom of the mattress (NBF, 1988). Heavier mattresses have a greater durability than lighter weight ones and price can also be a guide towards value. The non-allergenic properties of these mattresses are particularly suitable for people who are incompatible with the natural fillings used in spring systems (ibid).

Water beds are becoming increasingly popular. They provide an even distribution of support and are especially important for reducing pressure points for disabled people. Most designs require a heater to reduce the chilliness of the tough PVC; the heater is placed underneath a safety liner and is doubly insulated. A few new designs have sufficient insulation to avoid this. Most water beds rest on a wooden base but some are supported on all sides by springing (NBF, 1988).

With the vast range of mattress choice available, the final analysis lies with you and your particular comfort, providing the rules of support mentioned earlier are observed. Never buy a bed for its name or solely on recommendation. Test the bed for yourself. Lie on it in the shop, not just for a second, but for several minutes and test it in the way described below. Some firms make custom-built beds especially calculated to accommodate your particular weight and height. However, the best bed for you is not necessarily the most expensive.

Buying a new bed

- Take your time choosing – this is one purchase that cannot be returned, so do not hurry. Search around and test thoroughly.
- Make sure the base is firm. Bases vary from sprung bases with sprung edges to hard bases with slatted tops. The base is not likely to be too firm, but it can be too soft.
- Choose a pocketed spring or a mixed mattress. Enquire about the number of springs and test several mattresses with different quantities. Remember, the more springs there are in the mattress, the firmer it will be; the heavier you are, the more springs you will need to keep it firm.
- Do not test the bed by prodding it with your hand or sitting on it – *lie on it*. Lie on your back and push your hand in between the mattress and your lumbar spine: if there is a gap, the bed is too hard; if you have difficulty pushing your hand in, the bed is too soft; the bed and your back should just meet comfortably (*Which?* 1991).
- Roll from side to side. If it is difficult to do so, the bed is too soft; but the bed should 'give' to your hips and shoulders as you turn (ibid).
- When buying a double bed, lie on it together. You should not roll together. When one of you gets off the bed the remaining partner should not feel a huge change in the mattress. If there is a great disparity in your two weights, and you need beds of different firmness, consider buying twin beds that lock together (ibid).

Pillows

Most people tend to sleep on too many pillows. In any lying position the gap between head and bed is much smaller than you imagine; when lying on your side, the shoulder squashes round to the front so that the ear is much closer to the bed than the actual gap between ear and shoulder tip when standing; when lying supine, two pillows push the head too far forwards and can induce neck problems and headaches. One soft pillow is sufficient to fill the gap in any position.

Ideally, sleep as low as you can on one soft pillow, unless you have a medical condition which takes priority – a heart condition, hiatus hernia or asthma may require a high pillow rest. Also, if the thoracic spine has acquired an increased kyphosis it may be too late to change. You should do nothing to increase pain or discomfort, but you should experiment to see how close to the ideal you can get.

The softest pillows are feather or down, but if you prefer a man-made fibre, try this test: pummel a hollow in the centre and it should remain indented. Foam rubber is not good for this, as it resumes its own shape and never adapts to the contours of your head. A malleable pillow can be formed into a 'butterfly' shape, with a hollow in the centre and two 'wings' on either side; this allows the head to nestle in the centre, supported by billowing pillow on both sides. Sleeping prone (face down) is a problem for the neck, but it can be overcome by bunching up the pillow to form a slope against which you can rest your cheek on one side, with your face and your nose pointing towards the mattress.

All these considerations are important and they should, in the end, add up to a good night's sleep in complete comfort.

REFERENCES

National Bed Federation (1988). *A Selling Guide*, available from 251 Brompton Road, London SW3 2EZ, Tel: 071-589 4888.

Which? March 1991, Consumers'Association, London.

14. *Posture in lifting, carrying, pulling and pushing*

The prevention of injury

Lifting, carrying, pulling and pushing all involve conveying or moving an object or person from one position to another; they all place a hazardous strain on the body, especially on the back.

Large, obvious weights are not always the most injurious; it is frequently the insignificant movement of adjusting a patient's pillows or lifting a half-filled bag out of a supermarket trolley that provokes the back injury.

Recently, increasing attention has been focused on manual handling and lifting; with research applied in particular to the construction industry, the armed forces and nursing (Hayne, 1984). Many university ergonomic research units have investigated back problems in health service workers, continuing to seek out answers to the secrets of prevention: Does it lie in careful selection of workers, in diligent training or in designing the job to fit the worker (Snook, 1978)?

Selection: there is no proven strategy for identifying individuals who might be at risk in heavy lifting tasks (Robens Institute, 1986). Neither height nor weight are associated risk factors. The selection of staff is still a matter of subjective skill and experience of the examiner (Troup, 1977).

Training: everyone agrees that simply training people to lift and handle loads in a correct way is not enough to prevent problems (Birnbaum *et al.*, 1991; Robens Institute, 1986). The use of 'correct' techniques is often hampered by poor facilities, for example: insufficient space in which to perform the lift; shortage of staff, causing one nurse to lift a patient who ideally requires two; and a shortage of time, as in an emergency, when the need for speed supersedes the ability to think of the performance of the lift (Stubbs *et al.*, 1983; Troup *et al.*, 1987; Straker, 1989; Pheasant and Stubbs, 1992).

However, meticulous and well-monitored training is essential. Evidence shows that people can be trained to lift heavy objects in any position but they *must be trained*. If, used to lifting light objects, they suddenly attempt to lift a heavy object from a different starting position, they are put at considerable risk (Twomey, 1992).

Ergonomics: designing the job to fit the worker, combined with expert and well-monitored training, is the solution agreed upon by all references quoted. Following the European Manual Handling Directive of May 1990 (EEC Directive, 1990), brought into effect on 1 January 1993, new legislation, based on the ergonomic approach, requires employers to assess the handling of loads in their organisation; it requires them to prevent reasonably foreseeable injuries to employees as a result of load handling (Birnbaum *et al.*, 1991). Further information about sources of ergonomic advice is given at the end of this book.

The conclusion to be drawn from these reports is that no single factor is decisive. The Robens Institute Ergonomic Research Unit (1986) states that often the cause of back pain is cumulative stress which is then triggered into an episode of pain. Here we are looking at the triggers and the prevention of the triggering by promoting understanding and care.

The biomechanics of lifting, carrying, pulling and pushing

There are three main physiological and anatomical mechanisms for back support during lifting, carrying, pulling and pushing: an increase in intra-abdominal pressure; tension in the thoracolumbar fascia; and a combination of these together with the correct use of the muscles of the abdomen and back (Sullivan, 1989; Troup, 1979).

Intra-abdominal pressure is a physiological mechanism created by contraction of the transverse and oblique abdominal muscles and the muscles of the pelvic floor. During lifting these muscles contract involuntarily, raising the intra-abdominal pressure which then acts upwards on the diaphragm like a balloon, converting the trunk into a more solid cylinder which serves to support the spine by bracing it and transmitting the load over a wider area (Troup, 1979; Kennedy, 1980; Macintosh and Bogduk, 1987; Twomey and Taylor, 1987).

The movement can be performed actively by contracting the abdominal muscles to expel air against a closed glottis, a 'forcing' movement. This is known as the **valsalva manoeuvre**. It is used clinically to evaluate low back pain: it increases intradiscal pressure and tends to enhance pain because of the increased mechanical load on the lumbar spine produced by muscular contraction (Nachemson and Morris, 1964).

Intra-abdominal pressure is increased during lifting, pulling and pushing (Troup, 1979; Hayne, 1984; Sullivan, 1989); but it is greatest of all in pushing because the counter-pressure created by stress on the arms tends to flatten the ribcage. Breathing also becomes less efficient (Troup, 1979). This occurs less in pulling, especially when facing the load to be pulled.

The **thoracolumbar fascia**, described in Chapter 5, p. 65, comes into action passively at the limit of lumbar flexion or on contraction of the back and abdominal muscles. It stabilises the ligamentous mechanisms of the back, and by resisting flexion helps to maintain the equilibrium of the back, providing a major support mechanism for lifting (Bogduk and Macintosh, 1984; Macintosh and Bogduk, 1987; Sullivan, 1989).

The **abdominal** and **back muscles** interact in a complicated way to stabilise the spine and resist the force of flexion. They are a vital part of the process of lifting and it is important that their strength is maintained.

These forces all come into action during the conveying processes. In carrying, the time factor adds stress; while trying to maintain a static back posture intra-abdominal pressure will be held against an increasing tendency towards flexion of the spine. The biomechanical dangers are those of fatigue from static muscle work (Troup, 1979) and loss of fluid from the discs if the stress is maintained for longer than 15 seconds (Troup *et al.*, 1987).

The physical mechanics of lifting

In spite of understanding the above mechanisms there is still controversy about the 'correct' way to lift. This arises because the rules have to cover so many possibilities: the weight of the object, the position of the object, its cumbersome nature, the speed with which it has to be lifted, and how often the lift has to be repeated.

Lifting ability is a function of body weight, skill and experience as well as muscle strength (Troup, 1979). The greatest aid towards good performance is to understand the many principles of good technique and adapt them intelligently for each new problem.

One of the simplest ways of viewing a lift is to compare it with the mechanics of lifting using a lever, a fulcrum and a weight. This view may be considered unscientific but as a pictorial aid it is invaluable.

14.1

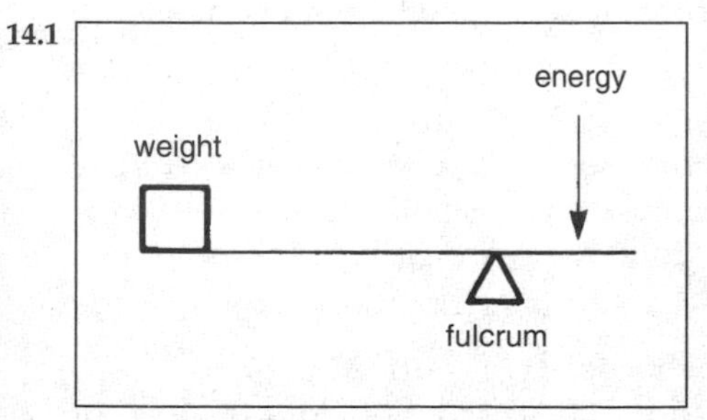

14.2

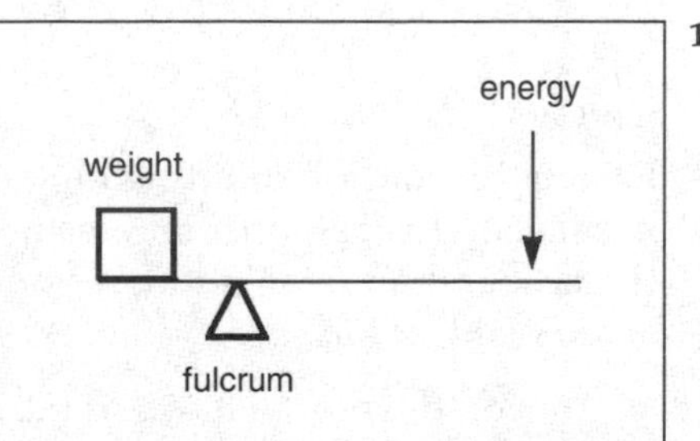

14.1 and **14.2.** The relationship between the fulcrum, the weight and the length of lever

Figures **14.1** and **14.2** show a lever, a weight, the fulcrum and the point of energy. In **14.1**, lifting is most difficult when there is a long lever between the fulcrum and the weight. In **14.2**, the closer the fulcrum is to the weight, the easier the lift becomes.

14.3

14.4

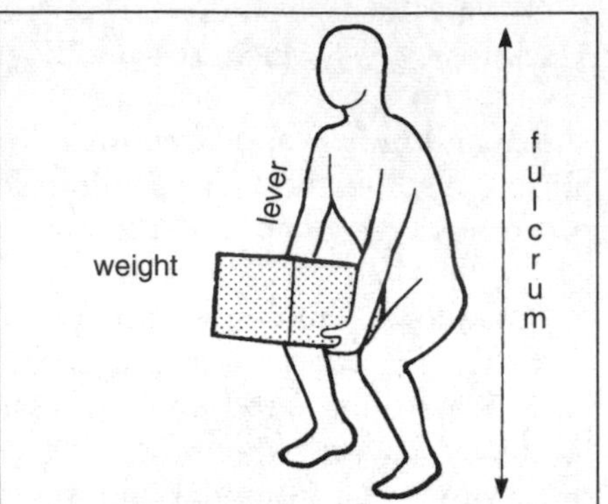

14.3 and **14.4**. The relationship between the fulcrum, the weight and the length of lever in the body

In **14.3** the *back becomes the lever*, part of its whole length from the hips to the hands; the fulcrum is at the hips and the energy spread over the whole back. As such, it is under the greatest strain. In this analogy it is not possible to move the fulcrum, so, to protect the back, it must be secured as part of the fulcrum, with the weight moved as close to it as possible, as in **14.4**; the legs, together with the braced back, provide the energy.

Discometric and electromyographic studies of the lumbar spine during lifting have shown that, in relation to changes in disc pressure and back muscle activity, the distance of the load from the body is even more critical than the choice between stooping and using ones legs to lift (Macintosh and Bogduk, 1987).

Guidelines for careful conveying

There are two landmarks in good conveying. The first is to calculate the move and the second is to take care throughout the whole movement.

Calculate the move

Each particular job of lifting or shifting should be assessed estimating all it entails. This requires an alertness, an awareness of the magnitude of the task and an evaluation of your ability to perform it in the best way, avoiding all risks:

- Are you fit enough to lift or move this object? If not, get help.
- Is the object too heavy for you to move? If so, can you split the load or decrease the size of it? If not, get help.
- Is the object awkwardly placed, for example a cumbersome weight on

the ground or a heavy load high above your head? The stress of lifting is greatest at ground level or above the waist (Liston, 1987). In order to minimise the stress in carrying the load should be raised or lowered to waist level before attempting to transport it. You then have the choice of carrying it close to your body in front or on your back.
- Is the object difficult to get hold of? Does it need additional handles or slings or ropes to assist the grip?
- If lifting is impossible, can you pull or push it instead?
- Are there any obstacles in the way once the manoeuvre has started, for example, stairs, furniture, uneven floor surfaces, difficult doors?
- Is it going to be easy or difficult to deliver into the new position?

Thinking like this may seem long-winded and time consuming when written down but it takes merely a few seconds in reality when you have trained yourself to think in this way. You may even do it in some way already without being aware of doing so.

Care throughout the movement

The position of the hands and feet and direction of exertion are important determinants of strength, strength being limited by the distribution of body weight and the extent of the foot base (Pheasant and Grieve, 1981). The position of the feet is vital; movements should take place inside the area dictated by foot position (Pheasant and Stubbs, 1991). If the lift moves outside that area, there is a risk of balance loss and decreased power. The basic principles for moving anything with your body are:

- Stand with a firm, wide, adaptable base in which you are able to shift your weight backwards or forwards as necessary, by swaying from one leg to the other, allowing easy flexion and extension movements of your knees.
- Use your legs to provide momentum and energy for the movement, so that your body moves as a whole.
- Avoid a dead-weight, vertical lift.
- Hold the object to be moved with a firm, comfortable hand or arm grip.
- Brace the back with a conscious effort (see dynamic abdominal bracing in Chapter 18, p. 193).
- Hold the weight close to your body.
- Avoid sustained lifting.
- Avoid twisting movements of your body (HSE 1992).

Guidelines for lifting

Lifting from the ground

- **Stance:** stand with a wide base, preferably with one foot in front of the other for surer balance. If possible straddle the object to be lifted. All 'correct' bent knee lifts, except those of the professional weightlifter, have an asymmetrical base (Grieve and Pheasant, 1982). Stand close to the object, feet firmly in position.

14.5

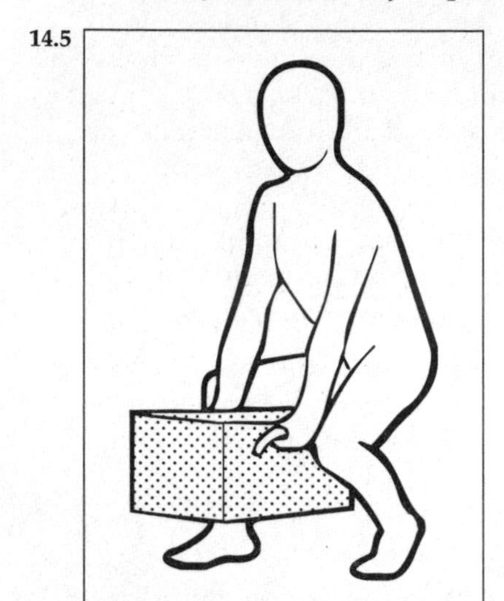

14.5 A wide-based asymmetric stance

- **Posture:** the shoulders should be symmetrically aligned above the pelvis, neither twisting nor bending in any way.
- **Knees:** the knees should be bent to the half crouch position if the load is not too low (**14.5**). However, if the weight is on the floor, the full crouch will be needed providing the knees are sufficiently mobile to reach the position and the quadriceps and hip extensor muscles sufficiently strong to raise out of it. An alternative method for the floor lift is to bend the back leg to a kneel position while the other remains a half squat in front. Floor lifts of cumbersome objects are awkward and require good training and care, or the use of hoists to help.

- **Back:** there has been considerable discussion about the position of the back in lifting, whether it should be maintained in a lordotic or slightly flexed position. The final decision is that using a 'braced' back in a straight, but not extended position, should be the first choice (**14.6**); that lifting in slight flexion is necessary at times and should be performed quickly; lifting in extension may require muscle training to be safe and effective (Sullivan, 1989). A full squat floor lift is impossible to perform while maintaining a lordotic back (**14.7**) (Sullivan, 1989).

14.6

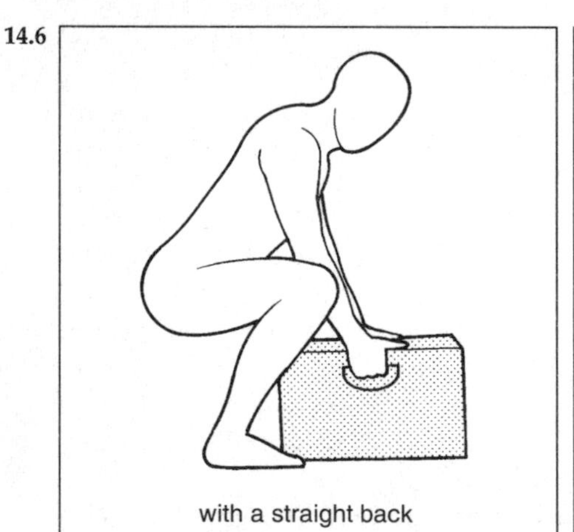

14.7

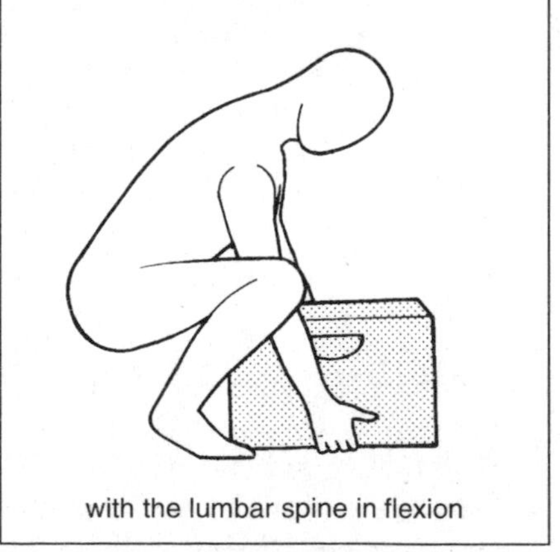

14.6 and **14.7**. The alteration in back position in a half squat and full squat lift

- **Grip:** grip the object firmly with a good finger/hand hold, adding a forearm grip if the object is bulky. Get the weight as close to your body as you can before starting the lift. Keep your arms close to your body. Use handles whenever possible.
- **Lifting:** lift the object by straightening your knees and hips smoothly, without jerking, keeping the weight tucked in close to your body.
- **Lowering:** lower the object into its new place by reversing the procedure: keep your back braced, bend your knees until the required position is reached and lower carefully. Do not drop it suddenly.
- **Mechanical aids:** always use hoists, pulleys, fork-lifts, or any mechanical aids wherever possible to avoid excessive strain; they should be used at all times when the weight is too heavy to manage, this applies especially to people like nurses, health care workers or manual workers who are constantly faced with difficult loads (HSE, 1992).

Additional guidelines

- **Always** complete the lift. It is dangerous to stop and hold the weight in mid-lift, or to suddenly change the direction or rhythm of the movement.
- **Always** keep your hips lower than your head.

Awkward moments in lifting

- **Lifting other human beings.** This book cannot go into the numerous techniques needed for handling and lifting people in the many different situations in which this occurs both in the health care professions and in looking after the disabled in the home. *The Guide to the Handling of Patients* (NBPA/RCN, 1992) gives detailed advice in words and diagrams for every kind of lift.
- **Cumbersome loads** such as full sacks: tip them up on end; try to hug them tight; use your body as a prop for carrying.
- **Long objects** such as step-ladders: pick them up in the middle; if you have to get to one end, balance the length of weight by throwing your own body weight further back.
- **Lifting with other people.** Make sure you are all co-ordinated, lifting together; use a 'one, two three, go!' to be certain.
- **Lifting from a shopping trolley.** Get close to the trolley, lean over with your back braced, slacken your knees and bend them slightly. Get a good grip with both hands well under the box or grip the bag handle. Keep your back braced. Lift with your arms as you straighten your legs.
- **Turning.** Having lifted the weight never twist the top part of your body leaving your feet still. Always keep your body in straight alignment and move your legs round in order to turn.
- **Lifting in or out of the boot of a car,** a baby's cot or at any time when the obstacle in front of you prevents free knee bending. Use the edge

of the obstacle itself for support, propping your thighs against the rear of the car or against the railing of the cot (providing the cot is secure). Always slacken both knees.

- **Fatigue.** Take special care in lifting if you are tired or unwell.
- **Clothing.** Beware of tight skirts, protective aprons or any clothing which may restrict the ability to move freely or the knees to bend.

Guidelines for carrying

- **Body support**. Carry all weight close to the body, even supported by the body.
- **Use your back.** Carry heavy loads on your back, for example, children, rucksacks, sacks of cement. Take great care getting them onto your back. Do not swing them round from the front in a twisting movement. Squat with the weight behind you, or lift the weight on to a higher level first, or seek assistance.
- **Equal distribution of weight.** If possible, split all heavy loads into two, one for each hand so that you are balanced. Pack two suitcases rather than one giant one for your next holiday.
- **Use conveyors.** Whenever possible use a trolley or conveyor belt to transport a heavy load (HSE, 1992).

Guidelines for pulling and pushing

Pulling

Never pull with your head close to the object and your back rounded (**14.8**). Wherever possible apply the hands to the load at a height between waist and shoulder. You can pull facing the object or with your back to it.

- **Facing:** your back should be braced; legs in a walking position ready to walk backwards. The arms must pull in a strong fixed hold with the legs doing the work (**14.9**).
- **Turned away:** brace your back; get a good grip of the object with your hands; lean forwards and push back with your legs (**14.10**).

Pushing

Never stand with your feet close to the object and, with a rounded back, try to push the weight away (**14.11**). Wherever possible apply the hands to the load between waist and shoulder level. Like pulling, pushing can be performed facing the object or turned away from it:

- **Facing.** Brace your back; arms firmly propped against the object; push with your legs in a walking movement (**14.12**).
- **Turned away.** Lean your back against the object, braced; arms by the side supporting the back; legs pushing hard walking backwards (**14.13**).

14.8

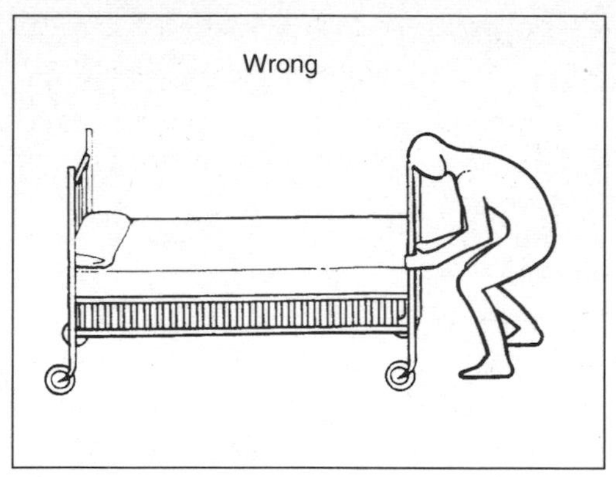

14.8 The wrong way to pull

14.9

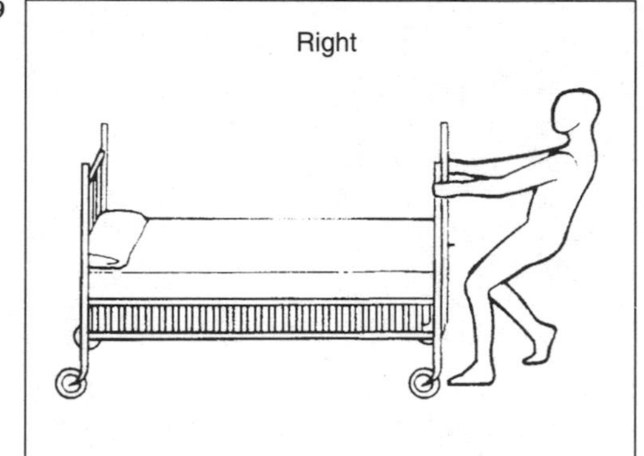

14.9 Pulling by facing the weight

14.10

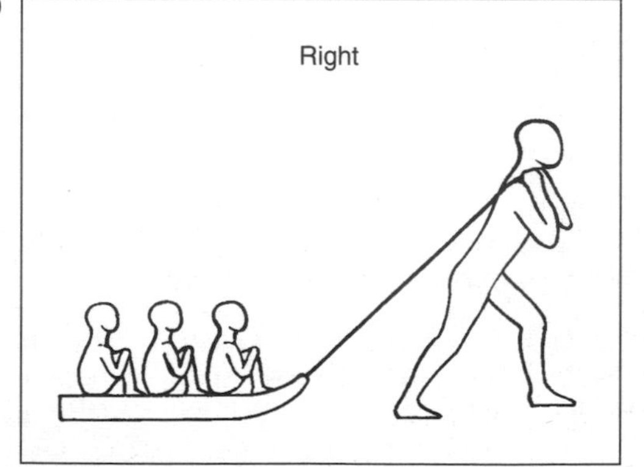

14.10 Pulling turned away from the weight, rope as above or held at waist level

14.11

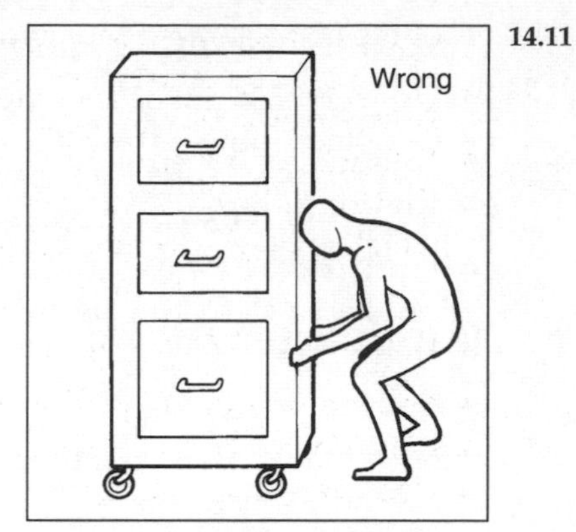

14.11 The wrong way to push

14.12

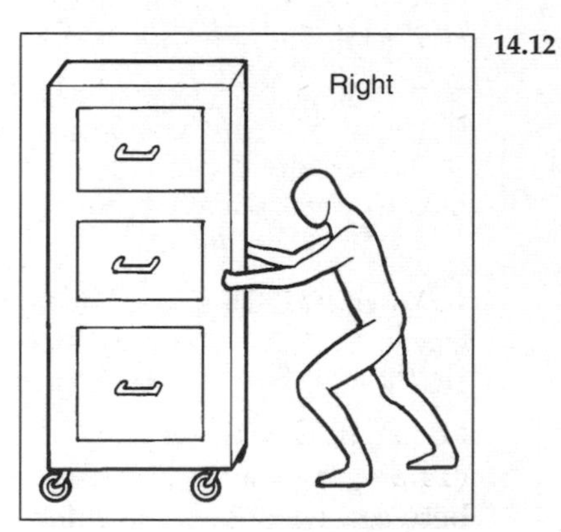

14.12 Pushing by facing the weight

14.13

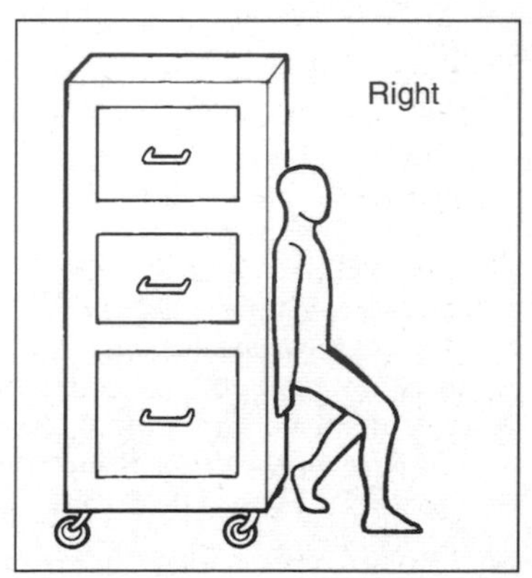

14.13 Pushing turned away from the weight

Awkward moments in pulling and pushing

- **Drawers.** Beware of opening and closing heavy drawers. Avoid doing so while sitting, especially if leaning sideways; always get up, stand well back in front of the drawer, bend both knees, one in front of the other so that you have easy free access.
- **Furniture.** Beware of shifting heavy furniture; try to have good castors on all frequently-moved items.
- **Floors.** Beware of slippery floors and a poor foot-hold.

Injury usually arises when the action is performed with the wrong force, the wrong speed, the wrong action or the wrong assessment of the manoeuvre. All these points must be given due attention.

REFERENCES

Birnbaum, R., Cockcroft, A., Richardson, B. and Corlett, N. (1991). *Safer Handling of Loads at Work – A Practical Ergonomic Guide*, The Institute for Occupational Ergonomics, University of Nottingham.

Bogduk, N. and Macintosh, J.E. (1984). The applied anatomy of the thoracolumbar fascia, *Spine*, **9**(2), 164–170.

EEC Council Directive No 90/269/EEC 29 May 1990. *Official Journal of the European Community*, No L 156 21.6.90, p. 0009.

Grieve, D. and Pheasant, S. (1982). Biomechanics, *The Body at Work. Biological Ergonomics* , (Singleton, W.T., ed.), Cambridge University Press.

Hayne, C. (1984). Ergonomics and back pain, *Physiotherapy*, **70**(1), 9–13.

Health and Safety Executive (HSE) (1992). Manual Handling – *Guidance on Regulations*. ISBN 0 11886335 5

Kennedy, B. (1980). An Australian programme for management of back problems, *Physiotherapy*, **66**(4), 108–111.

Liston, C.B. (1987). Back schools and ergonomics, *Physical Therapy of the Low Back* (Twomey, L.T. and Taylor, J.R., eds.), Churchill Livingstone, USA.

Macintosh, J. and Bogduk, N. (1987). The anatomy and function of the lumbar back muscles and their fascia, *Physical Therapy of the Low Back* (Twomey, L.T. and Taylor, J.R., eds.), Churchill Livingstone, USA.

Nachemson, A. and Morris, J. (1964). In vivo measurements of intradiscal pressure, *J. Bone Joint Surg.*, **46A**(5), 1077–1092.

National Back Pain Association/Royal College of Nursing (1992). *The Guide to the Handling of Patients*, 3rd Ed.

Pheasant, S.T. and Grieve, D.W. (1981). The principle features of maximal exertion in the sagittal plane. *Ergonomics*, **24**(5), 327–338.

Pheasant, S.T. and Stubbs, D. Lifting and Handling. *An ergonomic approach*. National Back Pain Association. (1991).

Pheasant, S.T. and Stubbs, D. (1992)(personal communication). *Back Pain in Nurses: Epidemiology and Risk Assessment*, Ergonomics Research Unit, Robens Institute, University of Surrey.

Robens Institute, Ergonomic Research Unit (1986). *Back Pain in Nurses. Summary and Recommendations*, Robens Institute, University of Surrey.

Snook, S.H. (1978). The design of manual handling tasks, The Society's Lecture, *Ergonomics*, **21**(12), 963–985.

Straker, L.M. (1989). Reducing work-associated back problems in the health service, *Physiotherapy*, **75**(12), 697–700.

Stubbs, D.A., Buckle, P.W., Hudson, M.P., Rivers, P.M. and Worringham, C.J. (1983). Back pain in the nursing profession, 1. Epidemiology and pilot methodology, *Ergonomics*, **26**(8), 755–765.

Sullivan, M.S. (1989). Back support mechanisms during manual lifting, *Physical Therapy*, **69**(1), 38–45.

Troup, J.D.G. (1977). Dynamic factors in the analysis of stoop and crouch lifting methods., *Orthop. Clin. North Am.*, **8**(1), 201–209.

Troup, J.D.G. (1979). Biomechanics of the vertebral column, *Physiotherapy*, **65**(8), 238–244

Troup, J.D.G., Lloyd, P., Osborne, C., Tarling, C. and Wright, B. (1987).*The Handling of Patients. A Guide for Nurses*, 2nd ed., Back Pain Association/Royal College of Nursing.

Twomey, L.T. (1992) (personal communication).

Twomey, L.T. and Taylor, J.R. (1987). Lumbar posture, movement, and mechanics, *Physical Therapy of the Low Back* (Twomey, L.T. and Taylor, J.R., eds.), Churchill Livingstone, USA.

15. *Posture at work*

Basic principles

Ergonomics is the scientific study of the relationship between the person and the working environment (Boyling, 1992). It examines the logistics of fitting the person to the task, or fitting the task to the person. Since 1993, in compliance with new EEC Directives (EEC, 1990), all employers have to examine the environment of their workforce, seeking and implementing the advice of qualified ergonomists.

Although this means that jobs entailing harmful stress will perhaps be avoided by substituting mechanical aids or redesigned machinery, it does not negate your own responsibility towards trying to achieve a stress-free personal environment. Examination of your immediate work space may reveal areas of clutter or obstruction about which you can do something.

The Institute for Occupational Ergonomics at the University of Nottingham has published a full report which deals with the workplace and surrounding areas with advice for full assessments (Birnbaum *et al.*, 1991).

The work space

Examination of the work space begins at the entrance: do the doors of the house, office, shop, hospital, ward, treatment room, factory open without undue force and, if they are doors for the public, do they provide easy access for all, including wheelchair users and their attendants? Stairs are a commendable form of exercise, but do they present an obstacle to the efficient transport of items or people within the building? Are people having to carry heavy loads up the stairs? Should a lift be installed?

Inside the building, is the room well-ventilated, with easily-adjusted air and heat? Heat, cold and lack of air can have an effect on the whole body. Is the lighting adequate and well placed for good visibility, especially for writing, reading, fine working and VDU operating? Poor lighting affects eye position which in turn influences head and neck posture. (HSE, 1992).

Is the furniture well placed for efficient work and unstressed movement? Are the storage shelves low enough to allow items to be reached without strain? Is there enough storage space? Are the cupboards and their contents arranged to minimise the time and effort spent walking backwards and forwards to collect items from them? If you moved the bedside table, would you be able to lift the patient more easily? Is there enough space to move the bedside table anywhere? Could the cartons that are always stacked by the window be stored out of the way? If you put the bucket at the back of the store cupboard, would it save lifting the vacuum cleaner over the top of it?...and so on...

Whenever you struggle with anything, stop and consider if there is a better way of arranging it or handling it or getting around it. Make sure your work is not made more stressful by surroundings you can improve.

You must become alert to the relationship between your body and the way in which you lift/carry/push/pull/manipulate all objects, animate or inanimate.

The height of work surfaces

Many work situations involve standing or sitting with a desk, table, bed, drawing board or some other surface in front of you while you manipulate and work with tools on those surfaces.

If the work surface is too low it becomes necessary to stoop, and the lumbar, thoracic and cervical spine are all affected; if the work surface is too high the shoulders have to be raised, arm position becomes awkward and tension develops around the neck and shoulders.

Standing at a work top: when standing, the work surface should be waist high or slightly below so that the elbows are bent no more than 10–15° below the right angle when hands are resting on the surface (**15.1**).

15.1

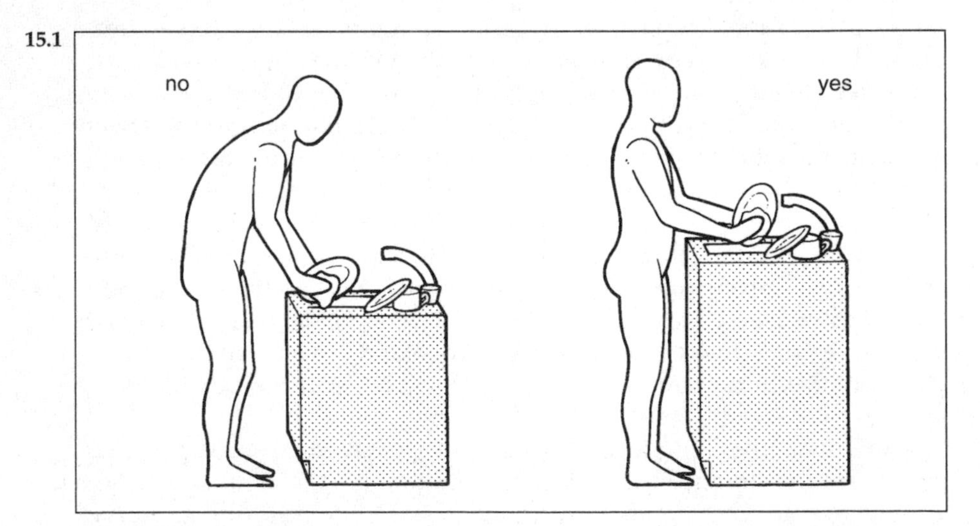

15.1 Correct work top height

Working at a bed or couch.: all therapeutic couches or patients' beds should be adjustable in height so that they can be raised or lowered depending on the need of the person administering treatment. The alteration in height should be performed electrically or by a hydraulic lever.

Sitting at a desk or table: if the table top is being used for writing or reading it should be at least half the height of the seated person (Mandall 1984). The flat top for office use should be high enough to support the forearms comfortably with the elbows bent to a right angle without having to slump forwards onto the desk (**15.2**, **15.3**). If the chair cannot be adjusted to meet these requirements, then the table should be raised or lowered as necessary. If there are objects on the work top which raise the level of work, such as typewriters or computers, the top must be lowered accordingly, or the chair raised to adjust to the required forearm position.

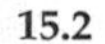

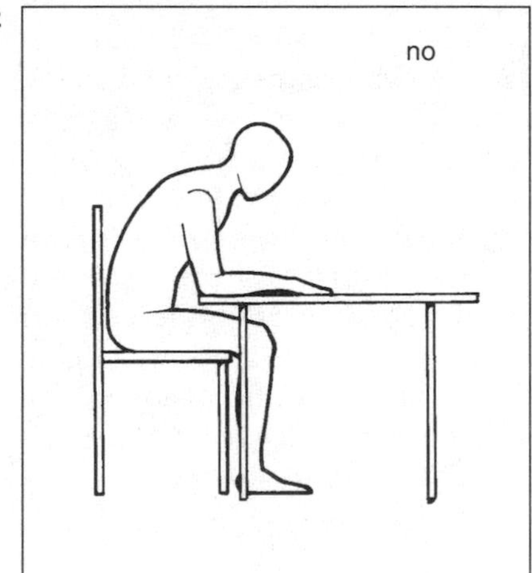

15.2 Incorrect desk height

15.3 Correct desk height

Sit close to the desk with the chair pulled well in to support the back. **Do not** sit on the edge of the chair and then slouch back for a rest.

Use an adjustable office chair whenever possible if working at a desk; other occupations which require chairs for short-term desk work or moments of sitting while supervising, such as nurses' work stations, should have well-designed, supportive chairs, possibly with armrests. See posture in sitting, Chapter 12, p. 131.

The slope of the work top

If the work top is being used for writing or reading the top should slope up backwards 10–15°. This is based on the fact that we tend to work with our eyes 30cm from paper or book (Mandall, 1984) (**15.3**). Portable, adjustable, sloping desk top stands for reading or drawing are now available.

The depth of the work top

No work surface should be deeper than the reach across it.

Work top objects

Accessibility: everything on the work top should be easily accessible. Implements on the desk, counter, kitchen surface should be organised in relation to frequency of use, weight of object and ease of operation. Heavy articles should be placed so that they do not need to be moved for easy access. Work out a good functional arrangement for all work tools, so that access to them utilises a variety of normal, free body movements with easy change of position. Avoid reaching for objects, especially if they are heavy.

15.4

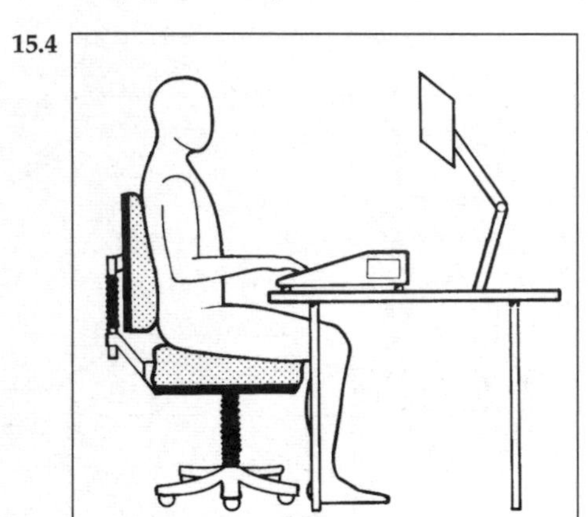

15.4 Correct typing posture, with a copy stand

Objects in relation to eye position: the position of objects in relation to eyes should be an important consideration when organising the placing of equipment on the work top. Looking at the keyboard, watching the screen, looking sideways at the copy, all have a direct effect on head and neck posture. All copy material should be on an adjustable stand (**15.4**), which should be placed centrally, or alternated from side to side every other day. See below for positioning of individual items.

Neck pain and headaches often originate from stress on the joints of the cervical spine after being held in either sustained bowed head postures or maintained rotated positions day after day. Looking down at work on a desk or looking to one side at copy work are typically provocative postures.

Visual display unit operation

The EEC Directive (EEC, 1990) has laid down minimum safety and health requirements for work with display screen equipment.

Chairs

All chairs must be fully adjustable office chairs with variable seat and back inclinations, and variable height adjustment (EEC, 1990). The chair back should be adjusted to a 90–100° backward inclination, giving good support to the lumbar spine (Boyling, 1992). Height should be adjusted to meet the requirements of hand and work top position, ideally with feet flat on the floor; alternatively a foot rest should be provided (EEC, 1990). The seat can be tipped forwards 5° if the operator works in a very upright position or inclined 5° back if the operator find this more satisfactory. Experiment to find the best results (Boyling, 1992).

Desk top

The desk top material should be approximately 30mm thick to allow for maximum thigh space (Boyling, 1992). The surface should be of low-reflectance and large enough to allow flexible arrangements of equipment (EEC, 1990) The depth of the surface from front to back should be 80–100cm (Boyling, 1992). There should be adequate space for workers to find a comfortable position (EEC, 1990).

Keyboards

All keyboards should be detached and tiltable, so that the worker can find the best position to avoid arm or hand fatigue (EEC, 1990). Keyboards must be at the right height for performance with upper arms relaxed and dropped to the side of the body; the elbows should be bent to a right angle so that the forearms are horizontal when the hands rest on the keyboard (Boyling, 1992) (**15.5**). The space on the work surface in front of the keyboard must be sufficient to provide supportive rest for the hands and arms of the operator, that is between 6 and 8cm (EEC, 1990; Boyling, 1992). The

15.5

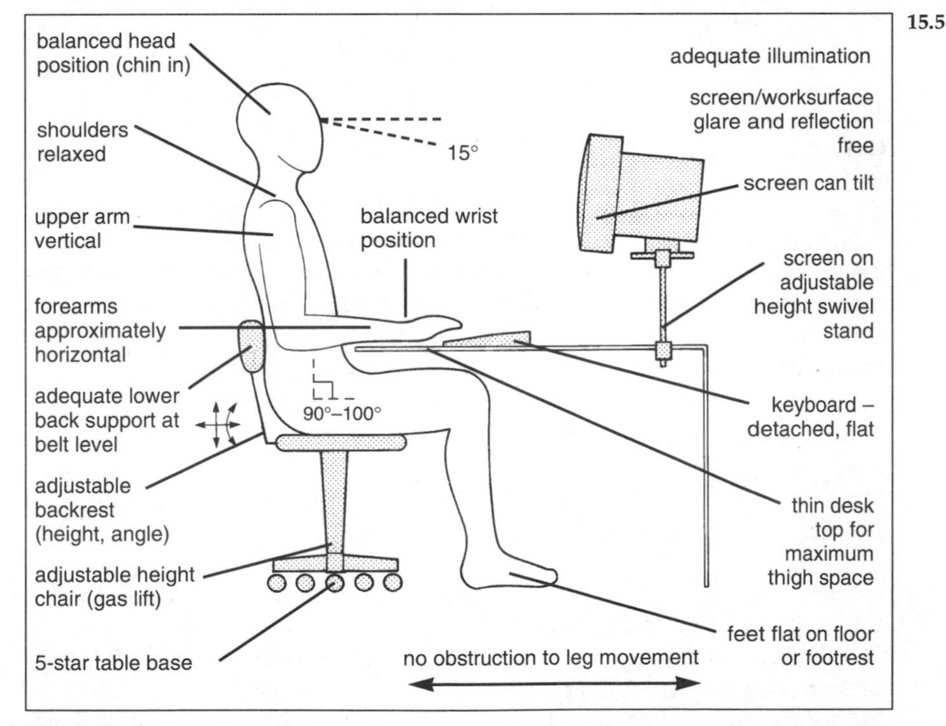

15.5 A VDU work station *with kind permission of Jeffrey D. Boyling & Associates 1993.*

symbols on the keys should be adequately contrasted and legible from the design working position (EEC, 1990).

Copy stand

The document holder should be stable and adjustable and should be positioned to minimise the need for uncomfortable head and eye movements (EEC, 1990).

The VDU screen

The VDU screen should be flicker, glare and reflection-free, with clear, well-defined characters; it should be adjustable in height, tiltable and on a swivel stand (EEC, 1990; Boyling, 1992). The top of the screen should be level with the forehead so that the eyes move through an angle of 0–20° downwards from the horizontal (Boyling, 1992). The distance of eye to screen should be between 50–90cm (Glazer and Glazer, 1991).

Lighting

The VDU screen should be at right angles to the windows or main lighting. This avoids reflection on the screen and protects the operator from glaring light (EEC, 1990; Boyling, 1992).

Leg room

There should be no obstruction to free leg room and there should be adequate space for change of position and movement. A footrest should be available for anyone who needs one (EEC, 1990; Boyling, 1992).

Work-related upper limb disorders

Work-related upper limb disorders (WULD) or repetitive strain injuries (RSI) are becoming more common, or rather, are becoming more recognised. They have been in existence for many years without medical diagnosis as such, many of their symptoms being part of other syndromes.

The symptoms appear in many forms but mainly as hand and arm pains or discomforts. They arise from postures in which the hands move slightly and repetitively while the head, neck and shoulders are held in a poor static pose (Cohen *et al.*, 1992). VDU operators are vulnerable, as are musicians who hold their instruments in set positions for long periods while their fingers perform.

The condition is avoidable by using ergonomically-designed work stations, by being meticulously aware of posture and by moving every 30 minutes, exercising and stretching all joints of the neck and upper limbs (Gifford, 1992; Boyling, 1992).

Office exercises

- Turn your head from side to side as far as it will go *slowly*. Repeat two or three times.
- Take your left ear towards your left shoulder, giving your neck a few stretches; then repeat the other side.
- Place your hands on your thighs, elbows by your side, turn your palms face upwards then downwards several times.
- Slump and arch, see 18.3 p. 195.
- Put both arms over the back of the chair behind you, arch back, stretching the arms down behind you.
- Clasp both hands in front of you, turn them inside out, keeping your elbows straight raise both arms with clasped hands right up above your head; hold the arms there and lean backwards over the chair, stretching your chest forwards.
- Put the palms of your hands together in front of your chest with elbows bent; press the bottom of the palms together hard so that you stretch your wrists back. Repeat several times.
- Hang your arms down by your side, elbows straight. Turn your arms with the backs of your hands towards the chair and at the same time flex your wrists away from you towards your forearm, then relax. Repeat several times. You should feel a stretch from elbow to wrist.
- Organise your materials so that you need to get up and walk around at regular intervals to collect essential items from other locations.

Nurses and other health care workers

The correlation between the incidence of nurses' back pain and the quantity of lifting that their job entails has been extensively researched and a definite link has emerged. The more stressful the area of work, the greater the incidence of painful back episodes; for example, nurses in general medical wards had a greater incidence of back pain compared with those in administrative work (Stubbs, 1982).

Later reports take this a step further, finding that, although re-education of lifting techniques seems to reduce the numbers of injuries, the improvement is not sufficient to place the solution solely on training, although it is vitally important (Robens Institute, 1986; Straker, 1989; Pheasant and Stubbs, 1992). Although an episode of pain may appear to stem from one particular incident, it is the cumulative effect of general postural stress, including patient handling, that causes the incident to 'trigger' the pain.

It is widely believed that nurses suffer back injuries because they are undertrained; the truth is probably much more that they are physically over-loaded (Pheasant and Stubbs, 1992).

The previous chapters of this book have emphasised the stresses all backs endure; the most common being prolonged stooping, twisting and reaching in the forward flexed position, frequent bending and lifting (Straker, 1989). All these are part of the daily routine in the work of hospital and clinic staff. They are also part of the routine in the domestic lives of those staff; this is a vital point. We must protect our backs during work but we must also prevent misuse off duty.

Ergonomic principles for the reduction of postural stress for the individual cover four or five primary areas in the system of health care: the equipment, the environment, the tasks and the personnel (Robens Institute, 1986) plus organisation (Straker, 1989).

The following list is a precis from the summary and recommendations made in *Back Pain in Nurses* by the Ergonomics Research Unit of the Robens Institute at the University of Surrey (1986), and published with their permission.

The equipment

- All equipment must be easy to operate and maintain.
- All equipment must be compatible with other pieces of equipment, fitting and working together.
- Each piece of equipment must be compatible with the space required for it.
- The equipment must be well designed for the task for which it is to be used.
- There should be good and speedy maintenance of equipment.

The tasks

- Tasks should not involve prolonged postural stress or awkward movements beyond easy reach.
- There should be frequent spontaneous rest pauses.
- *Task stresses* must not be increased by poor environmental organisation.
- Extra furniture such as stools and chairs should be provided to reduce stress.
- Nurses should be encouraged to choose equipment to optimise their own comfort.
- Sufficient staff should be provided to obviate the necessity of one nurse performing a task which should be carried out by two.

The environment

- The environment should allow for easy transport of equipment.
- The environment should provide adequate heating and ventilation.
- The environment should not impose additional stress, for example with poor lighting or unnecessary stairs and slopes.

Personnel

- Good design should fit the equipment, environment and task to the abilities of the staff.
- Nurses should not be expected, trained or selected to fit an inadequate system.
- Personnel should be encouraged to assess their own ability to perform a task, and seek help whenever necessary from equipment or other staff.

As mentioned in Chapter 14, *The Guide to the Handling of Patients* (NBPA/RCN 1992) also gives extensive instruction for nurses and other health care workers on lifting and handling patients.

Common working hazards

These common situations of daily activities are listed alphabetically:

Bath cleaning

Kneel by the bath or squat with both knees pressed against the side of the bath for extra support. Use long-handled brushes for the far corners. Arch your back to restore the lordosis after you finish (**15.6**).

15.6

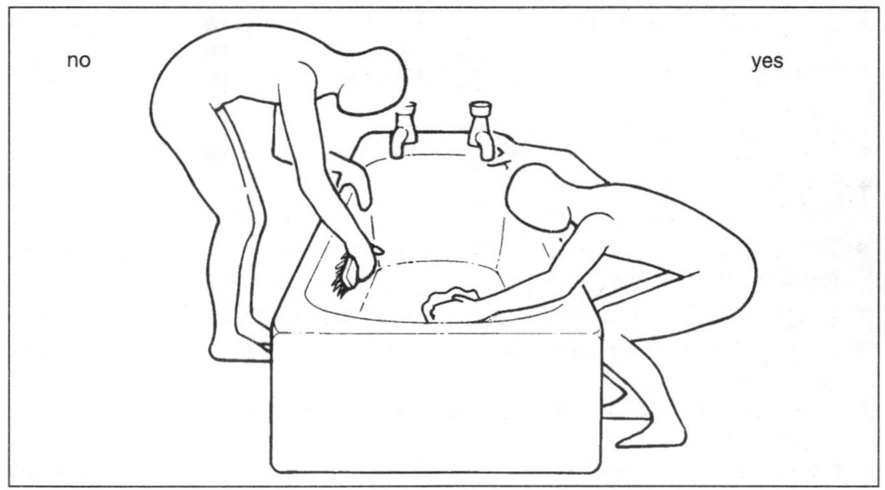

15.6 Cleaning the bath

Bed making

In the domestic household, either actually kneel by the side of the bed or, if this is difficult, bend both knees to half squat position and lean forwards with a braced back. Take great care as you throw up the sheets and blankets, this can be a stressful action. Duvets are a great asset for easy bed making and should be adopted by all back sufferers (**15.7**) .

In the nursing and health care situation, the bed should be raised to

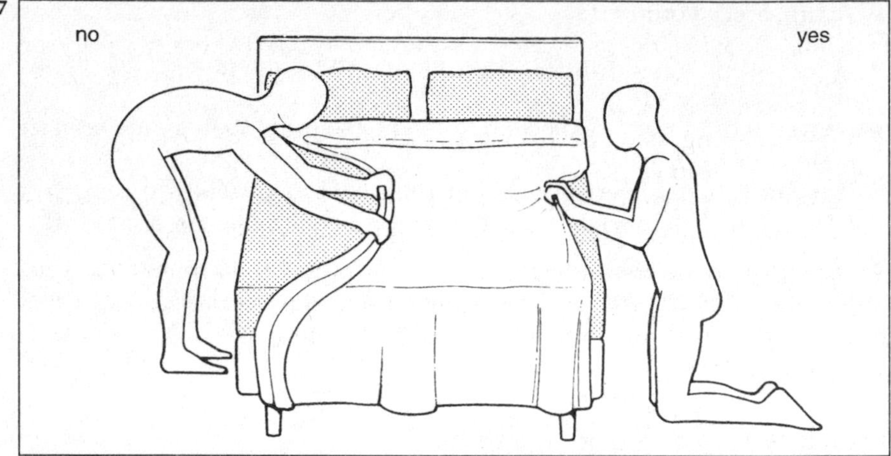

15.7 Making the bed

eliminate a stoop position so that sheets and blankets can be manipulated with minimal back stress. Two people should work together wherever possible. All beds should have good castors for easy mobility.

D-I-Y

- The height of the work bench should be adjustable for efficient, stress free operation. Use a wide-based stance for sawing. Rest one foot up on a low footstool of 10–16cm occasionally to relieve your back if it is painful.
- Take care when lifting ladders and planks (see Chapter 14, p. 153).
- Stand on firm planks or trestles when painting high, and get close to the job without stretching up. Avoid reaching while off balance.

Gardening

Gardening is one of the most common back hazards. However, with care, it should be possible to turn it into a good exercise with minimal risk.

- Avoid prolonged stooping. Bend your knees and get down as low as you can to whatever you are doing. If squatting is difficult, use a kneeling pad, or sit on a low stool. Stools on wheels are now available and they would be worth testing to see if they suit you.
- Use long-handled tools. Hang them up or prop them up when not in use to avoid stooping to pick them up and so that they do not become a hazard lying on the ground.
- Wear a pocketed apron for holding small tools to avoid stooping to retrieve them from the ground.
- Use a weeding box on wheels with a long handle.
- Take care with pushing. Use a lightweight wheelbarrow. Brace your back as you lift the handles.
- Take care with pulling, especially when pulling up stubborn roots.

Again, brace your back.

- Avoid carrying heavy bags, such as compost. Lift them carefully on and off the wheelbarrow. Remember your back is especially vulnerable because of the heavy work you have been doing.
- When digging, use your legs for leverage, not your back. Bend and straighten your legs as your back remains braced. Take special care with digging holes or trenches because of the twist in the bent position as you shift the earth. Move the earth only a short distance.
- *Restore the lordosis every 10 minutes.* Do not stoop to do something, then remain in the stooped position because your back feels slightly 'achy'. Come out of that stoop immediately and arch your back. This is absolutely essential.

Ironing

Adjust the ironing board to the right height depending on whether you prefer to sit or stand. A high stool is useful during periods of back pain. Use a small foot stool to change position and relieve pressure on the lumbar spine and iron for short periods only.

Kitchen work

- Work tops should be the right height (see work top height, above).
- Equipment should be arranged so that the cooker and sink are close together or, ideally, at right angles to each other, to minimise the carrying distance of heavy saucepans.
- Cookers. If you have a low oven, *do not stoop* to get to it; squat in front of the oven in a stable position. When purchasing free-standing cookers avoid the drop-fronted variety because the shelf, which is not intended to support a load, is a great obstacle to easy removal of dishes from the oven as it prevents you squatting directly in front of the oven (**15.8**).
- Sit on a high stool for lengthy preparations. If you have to stand to cut

15.8

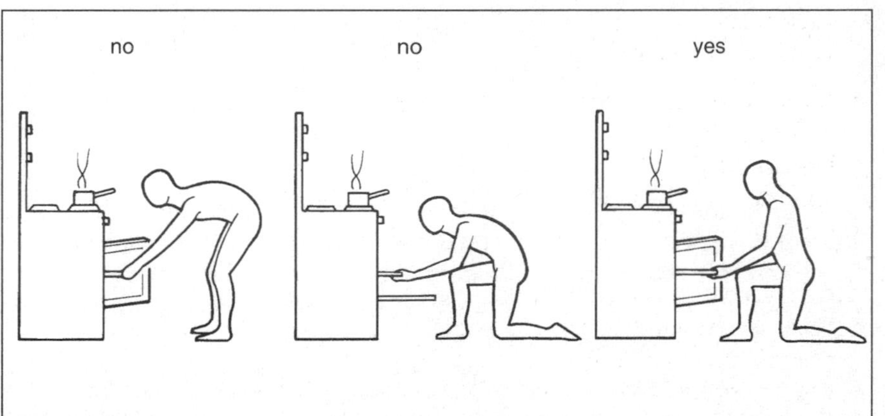

15.8 Using the oven

up vegetables or prepare food for a long time, arch your back frequently, especially your thoracic spine; this is where the stress develops when you are working with both arms held in a forward position.
- Keep a pair of steps handy for reaching into high cupboards.
- Use your knees when bending into low cupboards. Do not stoop.

Manual work

Although manual work is usually performed by fit people it exacts a heavy price in back problems. Read Chapter 14, p. 147 on lifting and carrying and implement the advice and care.

There are some insurmountable problems, such as how to protect the back when lifting objects into or out of a narrow trench beneath the feet. This is the type of job service engineers have to cope with when laying pipes in narrow channels below ground level. There is no clever answer. When you cannot get your feet level with the object you are lifting, you must squat as close to the ground as you can, preferably straddling the trench; think really mechanically about the lift and brace your back while you do it. If the object is heavy get two or more people to help, or try to use hoists and pulleys.

- Take frequent short breaks from work, restore the lordosis by arching and stretch your arms up high.
- Pneumatic drill working is another hazard. Both the stoop posture and the vibration are stressful. Stand with a wide, firm base, knees slightly bent and back firmly braced, taking frequent breaks with change of position and restored back arch.
- Remember the danger moments of manual work: twisting while in the stoop position, bending while carrying, poor lifting techniques, attempting to lift too heavy a weight, remaining stooped for hours without restoring the lordosis.
- After work, when you are tired, take care not to stand badly or slouch in floppy chairs. If particularly weary, when you arrive home lie prone on the floor, or in any comfortable position, and relax for 10 minutes.

Pregnancy

During pregnancy hormonal changes take place which soften the spinal ligaments, especially the sacro-iliac joints, decreasing their normal tension. Increased abdominal bulk adds extra strain at the very moment of vulnerability. Back care is extremely important, especially in trying to control the tendency towards an increased lordosis.

- Try to contract your abdominal muscles and flatten your lumbar spine. Abdominal and pelvic floor exercises are taught at ante-natal classes, so it is advisable to attend all classes that are offered. It is also important to maintain and partake in as much normal activity as possible, depending on any medical advice relevant to your particular condition.

- Avoid wearing high heels during pregnancy because of the indirect effect they have on the lumbar spine.
- After delivery, ask the midwife or physiotherapist about re-education of both abdominal and pelvic floor muscles – it is best to get them back to normal as soon as possible.
- In preparation for the new baby, be aware of the height of cots, prams, and places for changing mats. Try to plan all this beforehand. You need to follow all the rules of back care while at the same time ensuring the safety of the baby. Even tiny babies can fall off high, unprotected surfaces.
- When carrying the baby, keep it close to you, in front or behind. Baby carriers are marvellous but avoid using them for long periods; the front carriers put a strain on the thoracic spine and the back ones, though less stressful, can stress the lumbar spine. Try to avoid this stress by altering the position of the carrier and compensating with your own postural adaptation.

Reaching

Painting and decorating, construction work, cleaning windows, hanging curtains, reaching into high cupboards, pruning trees, picking fruit, and dozens of other jobs, all entail reaching above the head and reaching sideways. Stand firmly and symmetrically balanced, directly beneath the job (**15.9**) and use a firm step-ladder, trestle or table to stand on safely.

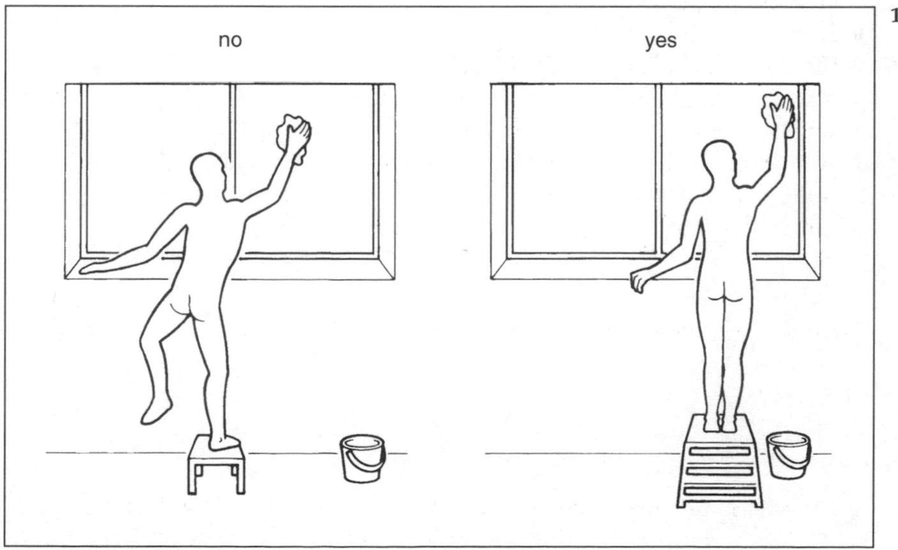

15.9 Reaching up

Sexual intercourse

Sexual intercourse is a naturally perfect activity for the lumbar spine, providing rhythmic, therapeutic pelvic tilts. However, it can be acutely disturbing when in a painful back episode.

If your partner has a problem back, have sympathy and use your ingenuity to try to work out positions that are helpful for your partner and satisfactory for you both. Fear of pain and fear of failure can wreak havoc upon a sexual relationship; the situation needs infinite patience and understanding.

There are many different positions to try, the basic rule being that the partner in pain should be the less active. Maybe you could start by the painful partner adopting the most comfortable position and the other trying to adapt round it. Possible ideas:

- One partner lying down, the other sitting upright astride.
- One partner on a chair, the other sitting on the lap.
- Both lying on the side, face to face with legs intertwined.
- Both lying on the side, back to front.

Stooping for small activities

These are the moments when we are often caught out, the times when we are performing automatically to accomplish insignificant objectives, such as tying shoe laces, picking up small objects, bending to alter a power point switch, and packing or unpacking a suitcase. You need to train yourself to bend into a squat or half-kneel position *whenever* you are performing any action below knee level. This must become a *habit* (**15.10**).

15.10

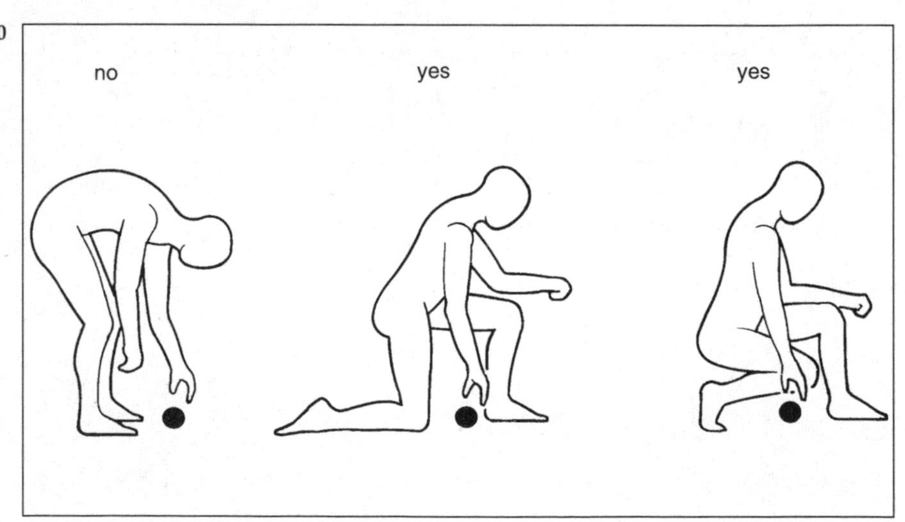

15.10 Picking up small objects

Vacuuming or sweeping

- Try to buy lightweight equipment at the right height and size for you.
- As you vacuum, slacken your knees, keep one foot in front of the other, bend forwards at the hips with back braced. Use small relaxed arm movements. An upright cleaner is less stressful than a cylinder. Restore the lordosis frequently. Avoid vacuuming the stairs with an upright cleaner, always use the attachments.
- When sweeping, pushing away from you is less stressful then sweeping towards you, but change direction frequently, sweeping in all directions. Restore the lordosis regularly.

Washing

Washing face or hair or brushing teeth are moments of stooping, and they are often morning procedures, which are particularly painful with a problem back.

- Ensure that your knees are bent, bend forward from your hips, bracing your back; if in a painful episode, sit in front of the basin, or sit on a stool if you are washing your hair over the bath. Better still get someone to wash it for you as you lean your head back.
- *As soon* as you have finished washing, straighten *right up* and restore the lordosis by arching back; *do not* walk around in a stooped position. If your back aches while in the stoop posture, coming out of the position *immediately* and restoring the lordosis will prevent the ache becoming a major pain.
- Remember that the early morning stoop is often a catalyst for the start of back trouble, especially if warning niggles of pain have been occurring.

General rules for posture and the use of tools

- Avoid storage in awkward places.
- Use long-handled tools wherever possible.
- All mobile objects should have good castors.
- Adapt your posture to avoid stress at all times, which often means using your legs and stabilising your back.
- Never maintain any position or activity for long.
- Change position and move around at frequent intervals.
- Always restore the lordosis immediately after completing a stoop action or a lift, or at intervals if the action is prolonged.

If back care is implemented assiduously in all these activities, abuse is minimised and injury becomes a far more remote possibility.

REFERENCES

Birnbaum, R., Cockcroft, A., Richardson, B. and Corlett, N. (1991). *Safer Handling of Loads at Work – a Practical Ergonomic Guide*, Institute for Occupational Ergonomics, University of Nottingham.

Boyling, J.D.(1992) (personal communication).
Cohen, M.L., Arroyo, J.F., Champion, G.D. and Browne, C.D. (1992). In search of the pathogenesis of refractory cervicobrachial pain syndrome, *Med. J. Aust.*, **156**, March 16.
EEC (1990). *Official Journal of the European Communities*, No. L 156/17 and 18, 21 June 1990.
Gifford, L. (1992) (personal communication).
Glazer, A. and Glazer, L. (1991). Sitting and the VDU directives, legislation and recommendations in seating, *In Touch, the Journal of the OCPPP*, **61**.
Health and Safety Executive (HSE) 1992. Manual Handling – *Guidance on Regulations*. ISBN 0 11886335 5.
Mandall, A.C. (1984). The correct height of school furniture, *Physiotherapy*, **70**(2).
National Back Pain Association/Royal College of Nursing (1992). *The Guide to the Handling of Patients*, 3rd ed.
Pheasant, S. and Stubbs, D. (1992). *Back Pain in Nurses: Epidemiology and Risk Assessment*, unpublished proofs.
Robens Institute Ergonomics Research Unit (1986). *Back Pain in Nurses. Summary and Recommendations*, Robens Institute, University of Surrey.
Straker, L.M. (1989). Reducing work-associated back problems in the health service, *Physiotherapy*, **75**(12).
Stubbs, D.A. (1982). Back problems in work and leisure, *Physiotherapy*, **68**(6).

16. *Relaxation*

Defining relaxation

'Relaxation' is a broadly-used term. Chambers Dictionary defines it as 'loosening of tension', which can be interpreted in many different ways.

'I am always tense if I am in the house alone'; 'I love to relax with a book'; 'A good game of squash helps me to relax after work'; 'I find it impossible to relax'; 'My shoulders go rigid when I whisk the eggs.' Each of these common and valid claims uses the concepts of tension and relaxation with different nuances of meaning. They fluctuate from describing an apparently emotional condition, (I am always tense in the house alone) to implying a purely physical one, (my shoulders go rigid when I whisk the eggs). A mixture of both is contained in every reaction.

Emotional tension

The most complicated source of tension lies in emotional stress, the body being 'held tight' in a protective defence for fear of 'letting go'. Problems which are common to everyone – excessive concern with work, difficulties with relationships, financial worries, worries of success or failure, can all lead to stress in our lives.

Emotion is an extremely difficult word to define because it encompasses so much. It involves feeling and behaviour, which in turn causes physiological responses like sweating, or a thumping heart, or physical tension like hunched shoulders. All these responses are the result of a situation (Strongman, 1979).

Anxiety is a natural feeling, one which everyone experiences at some time, if only before taking an examination. However, some people can become anxious at inappropriate times or excessively anxious over apparently harmless things. They may experience this anxiety when they least expect to, for example when they are watching a pleasant programme on television (Warren, 1992).

Inner conflict promotes a restlessness which excites physical tensions and results in loss of joint movement and pain. The cycle can become self-perpetuating and habitual. There are many typical signs of tension which you may look out for in yourself: clenched teeth and tight lips, restless hands, nail-biting, arms tightly folded or clenched fists, frequent sighing, perching on the front of a chair and toe tapping (Hare, 1986).

The key to solving these discords is awareness of the causes of tension and their effect on the body. It may take a lot of time to undo the causes of emotional tension but the effects can be alleviated by learning to listen to your body and learning to relax.

Physical tension

Contraction and relaxation of muscles takes place every time you move. Every action involves a balance between the two, as dancers and athletes know well.

Perfect posture requires continuous unnoticed interplay between muscle groups, when muscle tone holds and maintains the perfect pose; perfect movement requires a synchronisation between muscle groups with a quality of relaxation which characterises the performance of all great athletes, and is most difficult to achieve (Williams, 1979).

Although both 'contraction' and 'tone' must in themselves contain a certain amount of real tension, in this context, tension will be used in the negative sense, both emotionally and physically, as the antithesis of relaxation. Tone is a balance between the two. Many activities, like whisking the eggs, require muscle tone in some areas, fast contraction and relaxation in the moving joints and complete relaxation elsewhere.

Tension develops when a group of muscles contracts, holding a half-position for long periods, neither fully contracting nor ever relaxing; but the contraction is more than tone, it is tension. In this state the muscles restrict and inhibit the mobility of the joints they control, leading to stiffness and pain.

The beginnings of this tension may be a sustained position, rapid repetitive movements, or a poor postural habit. Tight shoulders while you knit, an awkward grip of the brush as you paint, contracting against the cold of a draught or seizing up as you trim the garden hedge, are all common examples. Neck and shoulder tension is a most frequent problem, and is often well established before being recognised.

The correction of tight shoulders is a perfect example of the need to distinguish between tension and relaxation in the body: as the shoulders are relaxed the tendency in the inexperienced is to let the whole chest sag and collapse back into a poor posture. What is needed is the maintenance of tone in the thoracic spine, opening the chest and stretching the thoracic spine forwards, while the shoulders are allowed to drop into a relaxed position. Performing this confidently needs a clear definition between the two states so that the whole manoeuvre does not become an either/or situation but a combined action. This is what the keyboard operator must put into effect all day. Only real physical awareness can make this possible.

So physical tension can originate from a postural state or from emotional stress. Whatever the cause of physical tension, recognition of it is the first step towards resolution. Awareness can only be achieved by being receptive to and in touch with the sensations within your body.

You need to evoke the sensations of tension and relaxation in the body and, by familiarity, learn to adjust them. This is what learning to relax physically is all about – to experience from within the contrast in sensation between the soft, floppy inertia of a muscle completely at rest and the alert, taut tone of one that is active, then to recognise the difference between shoulders that are raised very slightly compared with the loose, heavy feeling as they are allowed to drop, allowing the line from ear to shoulder to stretch into a long gentle curve.

We cannot monitor our bodily state all the time, but what is essential for good health, both mental and physical, is the ability to recognise the difference between tension and relaxation. We need to *know* whether a muscle is taut and ready for action or whether it is truly at rest. We need to *feel* the sensation which is peculiar to these two states. Similarly, our emotional vibrations must be discernible. Recognising the presence of relaxation and tension is the only way to achieve a balance between them.

Practising relaxation

Relaxation is not making your mind a blank. Quite intense concentration is necessary in order to learn to relax. It is possible to relax your mind while watching television, but you could, without realising, have rigid shoulders and crunched-up toes while you watch. Conversely, it is possible to be tension-free while you are hard at work, concentrating on a creative project. Reading a book or playing a game, (providing the competitive angle does not unleash other tensions), both focus mental energies. As a result they are mentally relaxing, but they may or may not be physically relaxing.

Physical relaxation is not a panacea for life's problems, but if practised regularly its therapeutic value is threefold:

- It provides a moment of stillness, a moment of quiet in the noise of disquieting daily routine, or a valuable regenerating pause in the midst of energetic work; 10 minutes that are entirely your own, when the jangle of nervous activity can settle.

- It teaches self-awareness, the ability to communicate with your own body. Many of us live inside the greatest stranger and we need to feel around inside the interior of the body edifice rather than admire the architecture.
- It is believed that relaxation, like Transcendental Meditation and some forms of Yoga, as well as autogenic therapy and hypnosis, induce altered states of consciousness, and decrease the activity of the sympathetic and motor nervous systems (Benson *et al.*, 1977; Melzack and Wall, 1991). This altered state of consciousness has been experienced by man throughout all ages of both Eastern and Western cultures (Benson *et al.*, 1977).

Benson *et al.*, (1977) point out that four elements seem to be integral to many ways of practising relaxation:

- A quiet environment.
- Decreased muscle tone.
- A mental device such as a word or voice or phrase repeated audibly or silently to oneself.
- A passive attitude.

There are several different techniques used for teaching relaxation which range from a meditative form described by Benson *et al.*, (1977) to a method described by Mitchell (1977) which uses contractions of one group of muscles in order to promote relaxation in the antagonist group, to a technique devised by Jacobson (1970), based on strong muscular contractions followed by their relaxation throughout the body. Both Yoga and the Alexander Technique teach relaxation in their classes and there are various forms of meditation, especially Transcendental Meditation which is taken from one of the Yoga systems (Hare, 1986).

There are many commercial relaxation tapes available from some record shops, such as W.H. Smith. It might be wise to borrow a few from the library first to see which ones suit you best. When you have found one that is helpful, practice it daily until you feel you can relax on your own.

Awareness of the difference between tension and relaxation is particularly relevant in an acutely painful episode of back pain. The common, and understandable, reaction to pain is to become petrified, literally; the fear of provoking a sharp attack causes a counter-productive tightening all over the body. The ability to control this by trying to remain relaxed everywhere, apart from those muscles necessary for precise movement, is one of the secrets of speeding recovery. This will become clearer in the next chapter.

REFERENCES

Benson, H., Kotch, J.B., Crassweller, K.D. and Greenwood, M.M. (1977). Historical and clinical considerations of the relaxation response, *American Scientist*, **65**(July–August), 441–445.

Hare, M. (1986). *Physiotherapy in Psychiatry*, Heinemann Medical Books.

Jacobson, E. (1970). *Modern Treatment of Tense Patients*, Charles C. Thomas, Springfield, Ill.

Melzack, R. and Wall, P. (1991). *The Challenge of Pain*, Penguin Books.

Mitchell, L. (1977). *Simple Relaxation*, John Murray Ltd., London.

Strongman, K.T. (1979). *Psychology for the Paramedical Profession*, Croom Helm Ltd.

Warren, E. (1992). Psychological treatment in physiotherapy practice, *Physiotherapy: A Psychosocial Approach*, Ch.27 (French, S., ed.), Butterworth–Heinemann Ltd.

Williams, J.G.P. (1979). Muscles, *Sports Injuries* (Williams, J.G.P. and Sperryn, P.N., eds.), Edward Arnold, London.

17. *How to cope with an acute attack*

Rest and care

The timescale for the process of injury and repair was discussed in Chapter 8, p. 101; it was then related to an acute back pain injury. This chapter reviews the practical issues of acute back pain.

The application of ice

In a hospital or clinic, crushed ice is manufactured by a machine; at home, frozen peas are an excellent substitute. They are better than ice cubes as they are malleable and more comfortable.

Take a pound of frozen peas, remove them from their tightly packed bag and place them in a larger freezer bag, labelled clearly 'not to be consumed', in case other members of the family decide to cook them! To make them into an ice pack, wrap the peas in one layer of wet towelling and place the parcel in another freezer bag to catch the drips, then use as directed below. Replace the peas in the freezer after use.

There are also commercially-produced ice packs, obtainable in chemists and some sports shops, which can be frozen and stored for times of emergency.

As soon as possible after the injury occurs, take the ice pack and place on the injury site for five minutes only. The best time for doing this is *immediately* after hurting your back; measures taken within the first 15–20 minutes of injury can make a difference of days or weeks in the time of rehabilitation (Knight, 1989).

Repeat the ice treatment every hour during the first 24 hours and continue if necessary for 48 hours (Ork, 1982). After 48 hours the length of applications can be increased. The guide to duration of each application is the reaction of your body to the ice. Ice should never burn or increase pain; if discomfort begins even before five minutes is up, remove the ice.

There is no proof that ice is beneficial after the first 48 hours, when the swelling will have decreased; however if it continues to give relief, use it less frequently for longer time (Black, 1992). Ice is used therapeutically in many sports injuries, given for 30 minutes at a time, every two hours or two or three times a day, over a period of several days, so there are many schools of thought about its application.

Ice should not be used on people with vascular problems, any person with a recent history of heart disease, or on those who have diminished skin sensation (Major, 1992).

Rest and care

Depending upon the severity of the pain you will either be working, with restricted activities, or you will be resting. The following positions and advice about movements should be implemented whenever necessary. For those on bed rest they are essential.

If you are resting, do not lie in awkward positions on the sofa, propped up in bed, or slouching in a chair. Use any relieving, fully-supported, relaxed position and avoid all provocative poses or actions. If any strange attitude relieves the pain when no other will do so, use it; just make sure that the strange position does not increase the pain after moving out of it.

Lying prone (face down) is often ignored by people in pain, but it can be the best position. If lying prone is relieving, it is a good preliminary position; you may need to start with a pillow under your abdomen, then, as the pain decreases, gradually remove the pillow and lie fully prone. You are then well on the way to restoring the natural lordosis. If this position helps, use it for five minutes every hour. If it increases your pain, do not use it.

Resting in acute pain

Figures **17.1–17.5** show possible ways of resting when in acute pain.

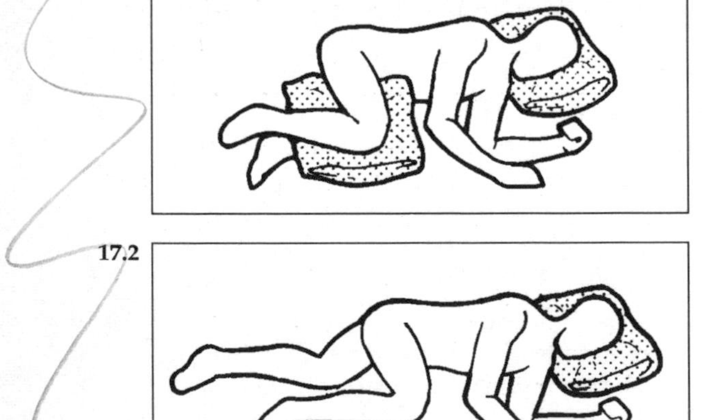

17.1 Lie on one side (usually the pain-free one) with both legs bent up and a pillow between the knees

17.2 Lie on the pain-free side with the painful leg bent up, resting on the bed

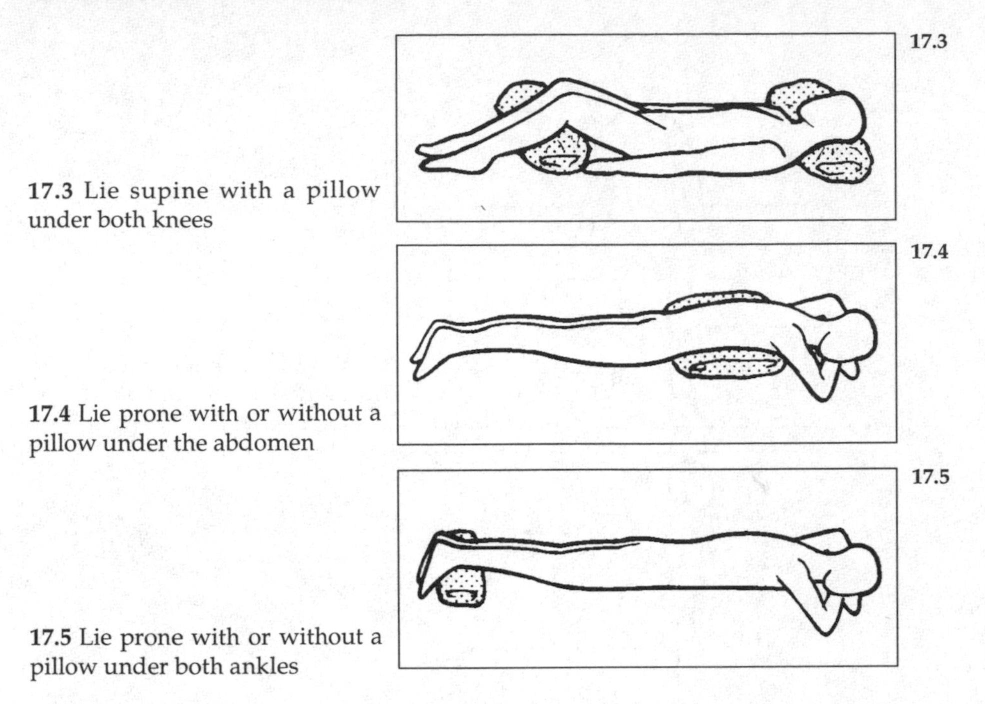

17.3 Lie supine with a pillow under both knees

17.4 Lie prone with or without a pillow under the abdomen

17.5 Lie prone with or without a pillow under both ankles

Do not stay in any position for long periods, because movement is good for tissues and inertia is deleterious. Change positions frequently but give the back time to relax in each position before moving out of it.

Rising from bed when in acute pain

Figures **17.6–17.9** show how to rise from bed when in acute pain.

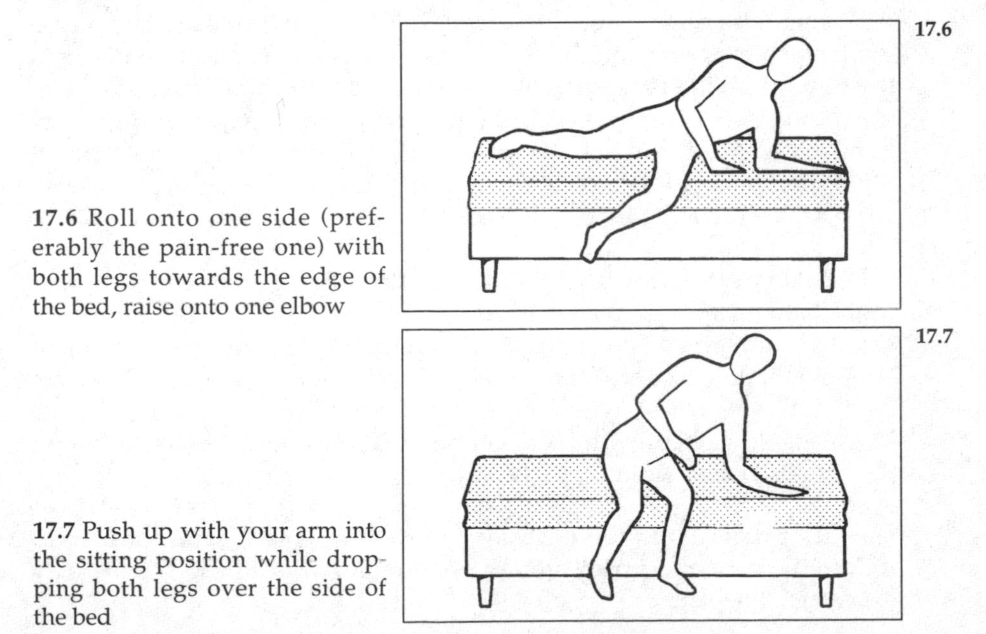

17.6 Roll onto one side (preferably the pain-free one) with both legs towards the edge of the bed, raise onto one elbow

17.7 Push up with your arm into the sitting position while dropping both legs over the side of the bed

17.8

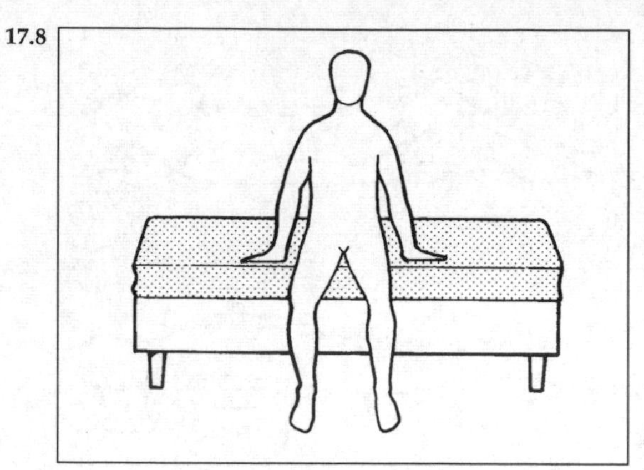

17.8 Sit for a moment and try to straighten up as much as possible

17.9

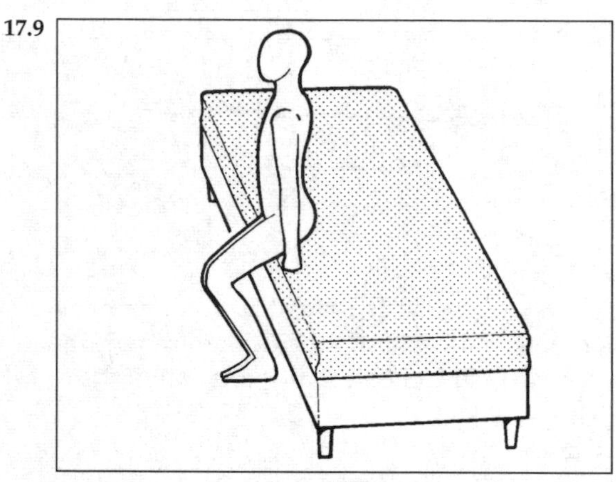

17.9 Slide to the edge of the bed with both feet tucked well in, brace the back, edge well forwards and straighten the knees

Resting with referred pain in the leg requires the same efforts to ease the pain by experimenting with different positions. The leg pain is from the back – nothing is wrong with the leg itself – so think about the position of the back combined with the position of the leg. For example, try lying on the good side with the painful leg bent up to waist level, possibly resting on a pillow which, if placed close to your abdomen, will also support the lumbar spine (**17.1**, **17.2**).

Leg pain may be increased by sitting with both legs out straight, either in the bath or up on a chair. This is because the lumbo-sacral nerves are sensitive and are put on stretch in this position (see adverse neural tension in Chapter 6, p. 82), and it is to be avoided as long as it proves painful. Sitting is best avoided if pain is severe, but whenever used, the knees should be bent with both feet on the floor; substitute a shower for the bath if possible or kneel in the bath.

Heat or massage to the leg may feel soothing but it will not help to reduce the pain; the very action of bending forward to rub the leg may exacerbate the pain.

If prone lying reduces the leg pain, use it. If it increases leg pain, *do not* use it. If leg pain persists or if there is paraesthesia or anaesthesia (pins and needles or numbness) consult a doctor.

Putting on shoes and socks when in acute pain
Simple tasks like putting on shoes and socks create a major difficulty; try doing these lying down on the bed on your back, bend one knee up at a time so that it is possible to reach a foot while the back remains supported on the bed.

Rising from sitting when in acute pain
Rising from sitting when in acute pain is a time when it is not only permissible, but actually necessary, to support yourself on the arms of the chair. Edge to the front of the chair with your back straight, put both hands on the arms of the chair, get the weight of your body as far forwards over your feet as you can and then push with your arms as your legs straighten, keeping your back braced.

When you are able to continue with work, back care should be implemented rigorously, with the least use of provocative activities such as driving, shopping, lifting, walking and stooping.

If **driving** exacerbates the pain check the backrest and the position of the seat. Use a lumbar support for the back and perhaps raise the seat by sitting on a sloping wedge or cushion. Stop driving if it continues to irritate.

After work, use pain-relieving positions. Stretch out on the sitting room floor if you want to remain sociable.

Recovery

After the first three to five days it should be possible to aid the repair process by gently increasing activities without re-traumatising.

Pain at this time is the body's Morse code and, if listened to carefully, will be the guide through the following weeks. In all activities, try to recognise the limits of the pain, learning how far movement can take place in each direction without increasing it – then use all the pain-free range as normally as possible. So, avoid pain, but do not over restrict activity and turn the back into a rigid pole, fearful of any flexibility. Rest after work and cancel all unnecessary social engagements.

Movements should be developed gradually into gentle exercises, the first being abdominal bracing (p. 194) while lying supine, providing it does not create pain . Progress into the exercises for pain relief on p. 194 (Kennedy, 1980). When you can stand and arch your back as in **9.1**, p. 113, do so every time you rise from sitting or lying.

Exercises should progress slowly to gentle mobilising movements, one or two at a time, increasing the range of movement as the pain recedes.Pain should be your guide for the progression of exercises, the important criteria being whether any slight pain experienced during a movement gets worse on repetition of that movement or lingers afterwards. If so, you are not ready for that stage of exercise. Never increase pain by trying to progress too quickly.

When movements are full and pain-free, the time has come to ensure that you are left with no residual tissue shortening; this is the time to start stretching each part slowly until you have regained full back and leg movements in all directions and to start steady exercises to build up muscle strength.

Injured tissues will never return to their original perfect texture, scar tissue always remains tougher and less supple than before (Evans, 1980). However, careful stretching remodels the collagen of scar tissue and should be performed, with attention paid to the sensations of the area, until previous range is achieved.

The average back injury takes six weeks or longer to recover, but can improve on a faster timescale. A severe back injury may take a year to reach full recovery and may require a full warm-up regime with stretches prior to undertaking any sporting activities for the rest of life (Williams and Sperryn, 1979).

The use of corsets

The old concept of corsets was that they restricted spinal movement and thus limited pain. It was later found that although corsets do not immobilise the spine, their compression of the abdominal viscera absorbs the stress that is normally exerted on the spine (Nachemson and Morris, 1964; Swezey and Clements, 1987). Corsets may substitute for the action of the abdominal muscles by compression of the abdominal content (Bogduk and Twomey, 1991).

Corsets provide a useful means for patients to continue with their essential daily activities during the acute phase, without unduly stressing the back. They are invaluable for people who find it almost impossible to stop work, such as mothers of young children. Not only are they a physical support for the abdomen but they are a reminder to avoid stooping during this phase and to use the back properly (Hayne, 1984).

However, it is important that corsets should not become a habit, they should be discarded gradually as soon as the acute phase is over (Hayne, 1984); the back must then be rehabilitated as above.

Chapter 18 covers the range of exercises, from pain reducing to muscle strengthening and tissue stretching.

REFERENCES

Black, N. (1992) (personal communication).

Bogduk, N. and Twomey, L.T. (1991). *Clinical Anatomy of the Lumbar Spine*, 2nd ed., Churchill Livingstone.

Evans, P. (1980). The healing process at cellular level, *Physiotherapy*, **66**(8).

Hayne, C.R. (1984). Ergonomics and back pain, *Physiotherapy*, **70**(1), 9–13.

Kennedy, B. (1980). An Australian programme for management of back problems, *Physiotherapy*, **66**(4), 108–111.

Knight, K.L. (1989). Cryotherapy in sports injury, *Sports Injuries* (Grisogono, V., ed.), Churchill Livingstone.

Major, K. (1992). Principles of treatment following joint examination and assessment, *Cash's Textbook of Orthopaedics and Rheumatology for Physiotherapists*, Mosby Year Book Europe.

Nachemson, A. and Morris, J.M. (1964). In vivo measurements of intradiscal pressure, *J. Bone Joint Surg.*, **46A**(5), 1077–1092

Ork, H. (1982). Uses of cold, *Physical Therapy for Sports* (Kuprian, W., ed.), W.B. Saunders Co.

Swezey, R.L. and Clements, P.J. (1987). Conservative treatment of back pain. *The Lumbar Spine and Back Pain*, (Jayson, M.I.V., ed.), 3rd ed, Churchill Livingstone.

Williams, J.G.P. and Sperryn, P.N. (1979). *Sports Medicine*, Edward Arnold, London.

18. Exercises

Defining exercise

Physical exercise can be defined as an exertion of the body in the form of organised play or specific movement which should promote fitness, be pleasurable, and gain in skill at every performance.

All activity is a form of exercise, especially if we remain conscious of employing all parts of the body without taking short cuts to make things easier for ourselves.

However, normal living, no matter how energetic, does not put joints through their full range, nor does it stretch soft tissue or regularly challenge muscular activity; for this reason it can become an abuse rather than a therapy. How many times a day do we bend our knees as far as they will go, or straighten them into full extension? How many times a day do we bend our backs sideways until the waist feels stretched? How many times do we run or move fast enough to become breathless? For many people the answer is rarely.

To ensure that we are fulfilling these needs we require a routine in which we play some sort of sport, perform a few selected exercises, or at least go for a brisk, stretching walk (not a stroll round the block) every day.

Exercise is necessary because:

- It creates strong, healthy bones, actually promoting growth in the young (Twomey, 1989) and helping to avoid osteoporosis in the elderly (Twomey and Taylor, 1987; Peterson and Renstrom, 1992).
- It aids co-ordination and balance.
- It maintains joint and soft tissue mobility.
- It strengthens body musculature.
- It increases stamina; there are strong indications that regular physical activity may prevent cardiovascular disease (Peterson and Renstrom, 1992).
- Mid range repetitive movements enhance the nourishment of specific tissues, especially the discs (Waddell, 1989).
- Last, but by no means least, it is personally and socially enjoyable.

Physical activity is usually associated with youth, but recent evidence points to an even greater importance for older people. The loss of capacity is often regarded as the hallmark of ageing, with an even greater loss of the body's ability to respond to challenge. Not only can exercises prevent many of the problems that have been assumed to be a normal part of ageing, but it also improves fitness and leads to an increased performance level (Muir Gray, 1987). Nowadays, there are many special exercise groups for the elderly in keep fit classes, Yoga, exercise to music and gentle aerobics.

Sport

Sport has only recently been accepted as an integral part of keeping fit; though it must be remembered that 'fitness' and 'good health' are not synonymous (Peterson and Renstrom, 1992).

The days are long gone when natural endowment alone was enough to secure success in sport (McIntosh, 1979). Training and practice are now a vital part of club activities if you want to compete seriously; and they are a vital part of sport for pleasure in order to protect your body from injury. **Training** means improving or maintaining physical capacity or endurance; **practice** refers to the repetition and betterment of techniques (McIntosh, 1979). One of the most risky practices is to play the odd game occasionally, with no physical activity in between.

Sport should be performed regularly, with good warm-up and stretching exercises before playing. If any particular part of your body is vulnerable, that is the area to which you should give special attention in the warm-up routine.

Some sports present potential risks which should be recognised, with the body especially strengthened or mobilised to protect from the stress.

Sports which entail stress in flexion/extension

Some sports include sustained positions in flexion or extension (for example, speed skating in flexion, gymnastics in extension) or high velocity thrusts into extension often followed by flexion (for example, serving in tennis, bowling in cricket, javelin throwing, high jump, windsurfing). These stresses can bring about substantial structural changes in the joints and soft tissues of the lumbar spine in adolescents and young people (Twomey *et al.*, 1988). Care should be taken not to overload a young spine.

Positions in **sustained flexion** induce all the previously discussed tissue stresses and changes: damage to the intervertebral disc by deformation and fluid loss, damage to the Z joint cartilage and capsules with stress on the spinal ligaments (Radin and Paul, 1972; Adams and Hutton, 1983; Twomey and Taylor, 1991).

Loaded extension or **high-velocity movements into extension** can cause damage to the anterior elements of the disc and stress on impact of the Z joints which increase the risk of weakening the pars interarticularis, especially in young people whose bones are still developing (Twomey *et al.*,1988).

Maintaining muscle strength throughout the body, especially the abdominal muscles and the back extensor muscles, is the best and essential safeguard against injury in these sports.

Contact sports

Contact sports contain all the hazards of accident and impact, and should be avoided during periods of back pain.

Sports entailing excessive vibration

Sports such as motor racing and cross-country motor cycling place stress on the intervertebral discs. The spine is subjected to vibration while in the position of sustained flexion, the motor cyclist having the added stress of handling a heavy vehicle. Back care, such as restoring the lordosis on standing after a period of driving, is essential; regular fitness training should also be maintained. Contrary to some belief, there is no evidence that jogging is stressful to the lumbar spine except in those with already damaged backs; it could even be useful for postural back pain (Twomey, 1992).

Sports entailing compressive vertebral forces

These sports include water-ski jumping, ski jumping and sports which involve high-impact landing. Research done on water-ski jumping found an alarming number of spinal injuries occurring in young jumpers, some only 13 years old (Stubbs, 1982). Measurement of the forces showed that the 'landing' force far exceeded the 'take-off' force but it did not appear to be intense enough to injure normal, healthy adult spines. However, the report suggest an urgent review and limitation of jumping for adolescents, possibly by reducing the jump heights, or the boat speed, or by restricting the events to people over 16 years of age (ibid).

Water sports

Swimming is the ideal sport for back sufferers: the action is performed in a non-weight bearing position for the spine, with water giving full support. Considerable movement takes place in the back, arms and legs and the movement can be varied with frequent changes of stroke. Swimming can be performed as gently or as energetically as desired, and can be used aerobically by speeding up the pace. Aquarobics (exercises in water) is becoming more and more popular, especially for the elderly and offers a mode of good all-round rehabilitation (Baum, 1991).

Every sport has its risk element – the aim of investigating these is not to deter people from participating but to make the activity safer (Stubbs, 1982). A comprehensive evaluation of the risk to the back of every sport would fill another book.

Many joint injuries are preventable by accurate basic training to condition the joint, understanding the role of the joint in the sport to be performed, developing adequate muscle strength for the task, and meticulous attention to technique training (Thomason, 1979).

Providing you have no back problems, choose a sport you want to play, get the best advice about training for it, train carefully and play regularly. If you are a casual sports player, make sure you keep your body fit with regular exercises, especially for your back and abdominal muscles.

If you have back problems consult a sports medical practitioner or sports physiotherapist who should be able to give advice about your best mode of rehabilitation.

Exercising

Useful terminology

Specific terms are used to describe and abbreviate the description of certain exercise starting positions:

Supine: lying on the back
Prone: lying face downwards
Crook lying: lying on the back with both knees bent and both feet on the floor
Prone kneeling: kneeling on all fours in a crawling position

Criteria for pain during exercise

Without a full examination it is impossible to say which exercises are best for any person, especially for someone who has recently had a period of back pain. I can therefore only give you guidance about exercises for pain, and emphasise that no exercise should be performed either because it appears here, because you feel it *ought* to be done, or because someone else you know is doing it with good results.

- If you experience sharp, severe or lasting pain during any exercise – *stop and do not repeat it*.
- If you feel slight pain which occurs while pushing into the end of range of any movement but which goes as soon as the over-pressure is released, and which does not elicit pain later, the pain is probably

related to the stretching of tight tissue and should gradually lessen with repetition of the movement. If this is so, the exercise can be continued and the range of movement should gradually increase.
- If you experience pain after exercising, try to analyse whether it is a muscular pain from muscular fatigue or an increase of your original pain: if the former, the exercise can be repeated but not progressed until the muscles stop reacting; if it is an increase of your pain either repeat less vigorously, or with fewer repetitions, or stop the exercise if in doubt.
- Introduce one new exercise at a time so that you can monitor the effect of each.
- *Do not* persevere with any exercise which gives lasting pain after performance.

This book looks at therapeutic exercises, exercises for mobilising the joints of the spine, for strengthening and stabilising the muscles of the trunk, for correcting a thoracic kyphosis and 'poking chin', exercises for stretching the hips and knees and exercises for endurance.

Each section begins with easier exercises. If you are pain free, aim to build up a routine with one or two exercises from each section. If you are recovering from a painful episode choose only one exercise until you are confident that there is no increase of pain, then add another from a different section and so on, respecting the criteria for exercises in relation to pain. You need no more than six exercises in any one regime. Start with the minimum number of repetitions and increase only when you feel you can.

Therapeutic exercises

Therapeutic exercises are designed to aid specific problems. Providing a universal routine without assessment of any individual pain is impossible. In the past there were two opposing schools of thought, one advocating flexion and the other advocating extension as the method to reduce pain and re-educate the back. Success was haphazard.

The question of which movement to use for your pain must be answered by the response of your tissues to the movement.

McKenzie exercises: Robin McKenzie, a consultant in spinal therapy in New Zealand, has worked out a principle of examination of spinal problems, using repeated movements, which are in themselves diagnostic; the exercises can then be used therapeutically. His principles are described in two excellent books which are available in the United Kingdom, *Treat Your Own Back* and *Treat Your Own Neck*. Read them carefully – some people manage to do the wrong thing in spite of McKenzie's clear step-by-step instructions!

Back bracing or dynamic abdominal bracing (DAB)

Back bracing or dynamic abdominal bracing is the manoeuvre which utilises the intra-abdominal pressure mechanism to stabilise and protect the lumbar spine during movements in weight bearing (Kennedy, 1980).

Practise the procedure in standing. place your hands on your hips, just above the iliac crests with your fingers resting on the muscles at the side of the abdomen. Make a forcing down movement inside your abdomen and at the same time contract the abdominal muscles where your hands are to control or counteract this forcing pressure; go on breathing. Do not hollow your abdomen. Do not push your abdomen out. Hold for a count of 10. While you maintain this forcing hold, the glottis should not be closed. Air should travel freely in and out. There should be no feelings of head pressure (Kennedy, 1980). The oblique and transverse abdominals are doing the work.

This is the 'back bracing' movement referred to in all lifting. It is one of the abdominal exercises mentioned on p. 201 and it can be used as the first exercise to start during anuy acute episode of back pain (Kennedy, 1980). Used in this way it should be practised in crook lying to start with and performed within the limits of your pain.

As soon as dynamic abdominal bracing can be performed without pain, use it for exercising:

- Crook lying, brace, hold, and breathe while you hold for a count of five, then relax. Repeat 4–5 times.
- Crook lying, lift one knee towards the chest, place both hands around the knee, brace, pull slightly on the knee to increase the brace, then relax. Repeat with the other leg. Repeat 4–5 times.
- Crook lying, put both hands behind the waist, brace, then push the lumbar spine back onto the hands, relax. Repeat 4–5 times (Kennedy, 1980).

These exercises should not be performed if they increase pain in any way. If they help to decrease pain, the length of 'hold' and the number of repetitions can be gradually increased. They should not increase head pressure.

Exercises for mobility

Flexion and extension

Many of the mobilising exercises here use both movements of flexion/extension alternately. If stiffness is your problem rather than pain, use both movements as described; if one of these movements gives you pain, do not push into it, use the pain-free movement while just moving slightly into the other in a pain-free range. Choose the movements that you feel are right for your particular needs.

18.1 Crook lying, pull both knees up towards the chest, clasp a hand round each knee and pull up to your chest, allowing your buttocks to leave the floor. Lower your feet back onto the floor. Do this 5–10 times (McKenzie, 1981).

18.1

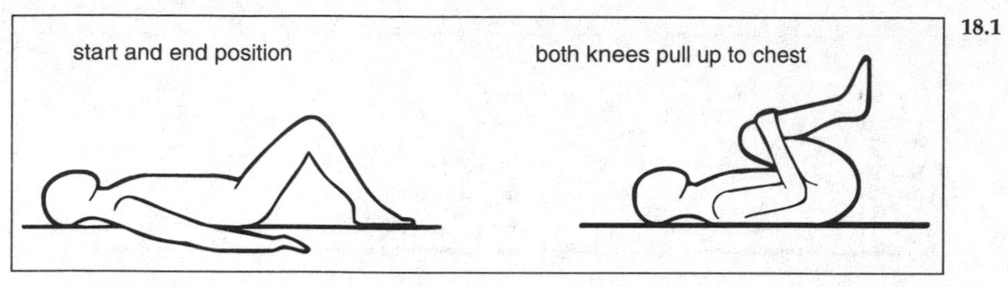

18.1 Passive lumbar flexion

18.2 Prone lying, place your hands on the floor by your shoulders, push with your arms and raise your shoulders passively right off the ground, as high as you can push without pain, if possible until your arms are straight. It is *essential* that your shoulders, back and buttocks *remain completely relaxed* while your arms do all the work. Lower back to the starting position. Repeat 5–10 times. (McKenzie, 1981)

18.2

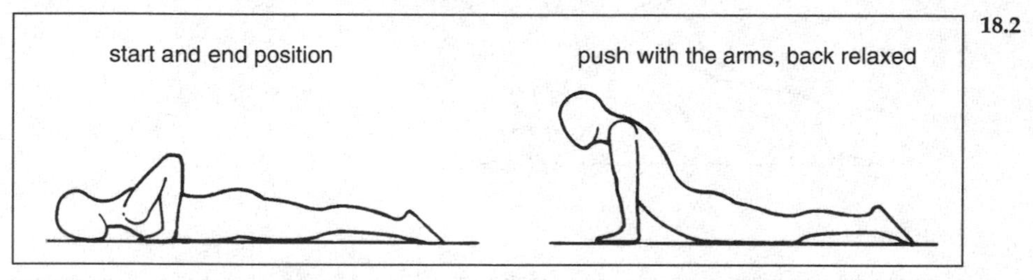

18.2 Passive lumbar extension

18.3 Sitting on a stool, slump your back into a relaxed round, pull your head down on to your chest, then arch back, retracting your chin as you do so. Repeat 3–4 times. This is a movement that may be painful for those people recovering from a back condition, so use only part of it, or use it very gently until your back gains in pain-free mobility.

18.3

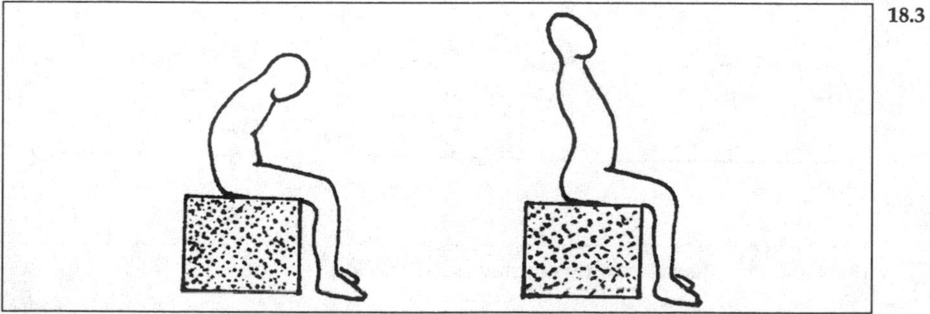

18.3 Slump and arch

18.4 Prone kneeling, with your arms and thighs forming a rectangle, hump and hollow your back in an easy, repetitive movement. Keep your arms straight and your legs steady, do not sway backwards and forwards. Repeat 5–10 times.

18.4

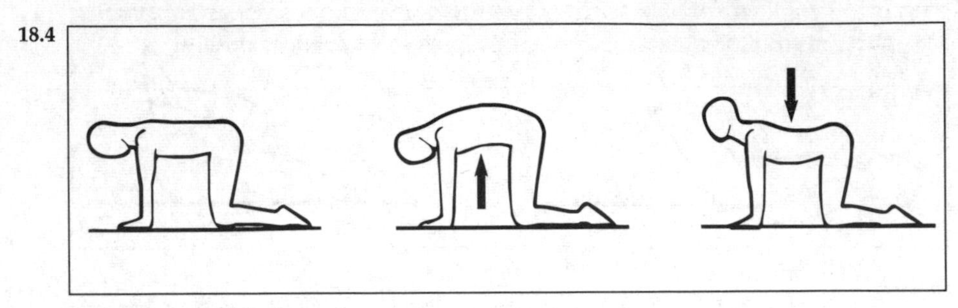

18.4 Hump and hollow

18.5 Crook lying, lift your hips off the floor as high as you can, hollow your abdomen and tighten your buttocks. Hold for a count of 10, then lower. Repeat 5–10 times.

18.5

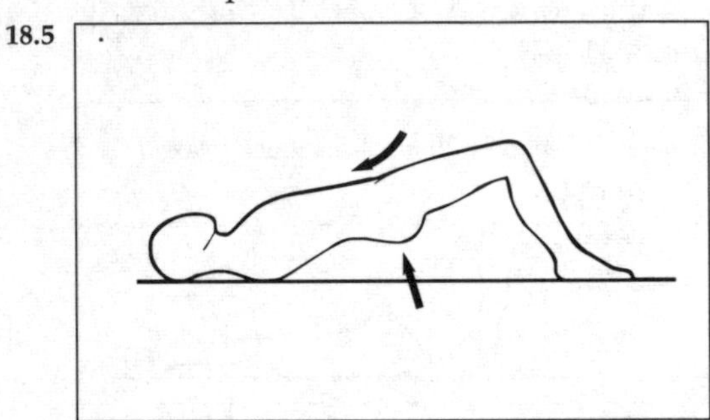

18.5 Bridging

18.6 Prone kneeling, tuck your head towards your chest and pull one knee under towards your forehead, then straighten the leg out backwards to the level of your buttocks lifting your head at the same time. Repeat with the other leg. Repeat 5–10 times.

18.6

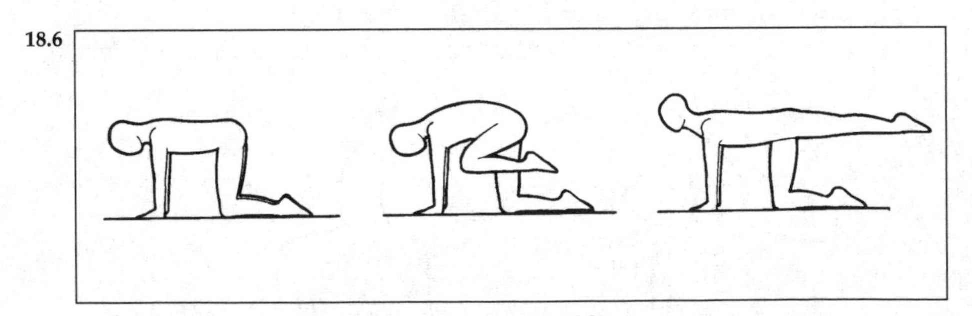

18.6 Flexion/extension exercise using head and leg

Exercises **18.7, 18 8 – 18.9** target the thoracic spine: **18.8** and **18.9** have the same movement but use different methods of stabilising the pelvis:

18.7 Kneeling, sitting back on your heels and leaning forwards onto your forearms: tuck your head under towards your knees, then raise your head high and let your shoulders drop. Repeat 3–6 times, slowly.

18.7

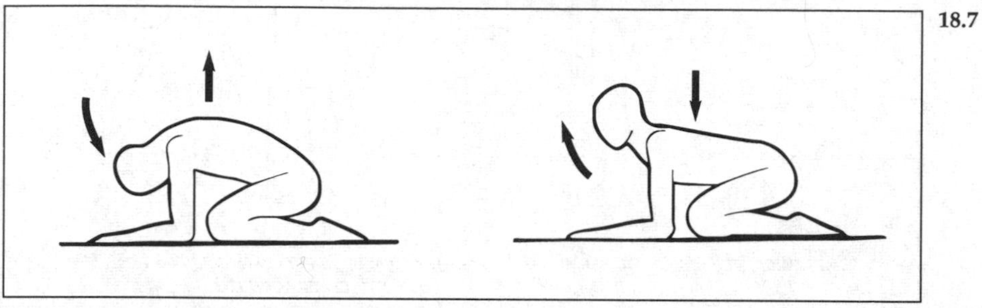

18.7 Thoracic spine flexion/extension

18.8 Kneel on the floor with your arms outstretched in front of you, holding on to the back of a chair. Keep your legs and pelvis still, arch your chest forwards towards the back of the chair, then relax. Repeat 3–5 times.

18.8

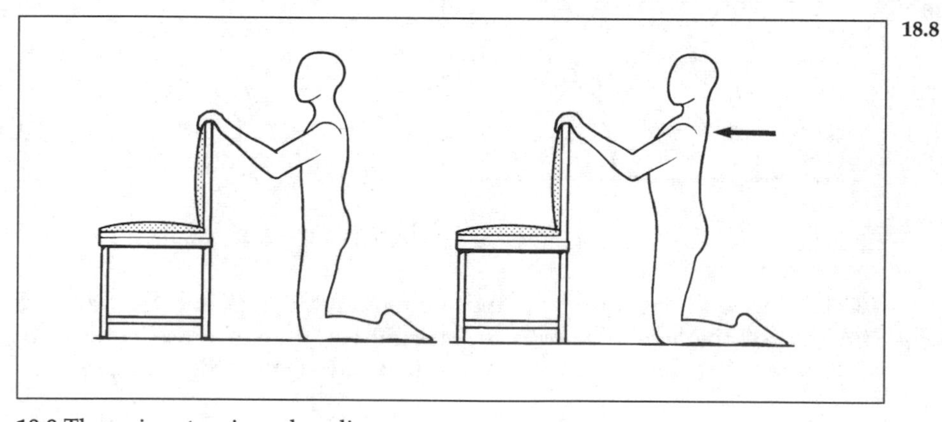

18.8 Thoracic extension – kneeling

18.9 Stand by a high table, almost touching it with your hips, stand up straight so that your legs are vertical, making sure that you are not swaying forwards at the hips; arch your chest forwards without allowing your hips to press on or move towards the table, hold, and try to feel the movement. Repeat slowly 3–5 times.

18.9

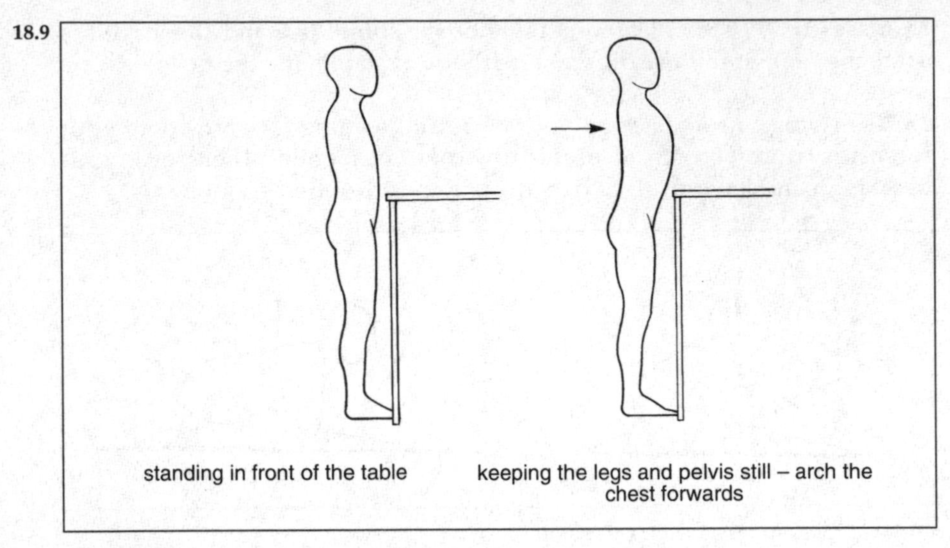

18.9 Thoracic extension – standing

Rotation

18.10 Crook lying, roll both knees as far as you can one way and then roll to the other, trying gradually to increase the range. Repeat 10 times.

18.10

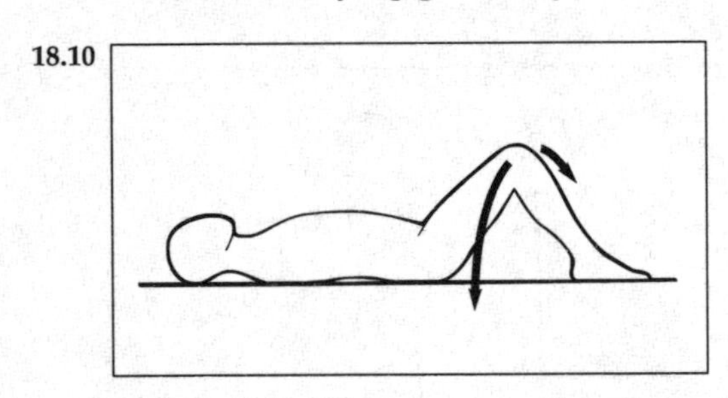

18.10 Double knee rolling

18.11 Lying with one knee bent and the foot on the floor and the other leg straight: roll the bent knee over the straight leg, press it towards the floor and bring it up again. Repeat 4–6 times. Repeat with the other knee.

18.11

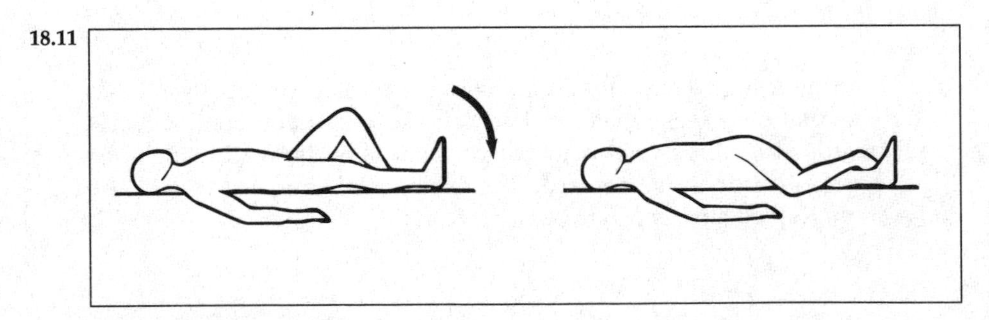

18.11 Single knee rolling

18.12 Lying supine, pull both knees up towards your chest, hold them up and roll both knees from side to side, touching the floor if you can. Repeat 5–6 times.

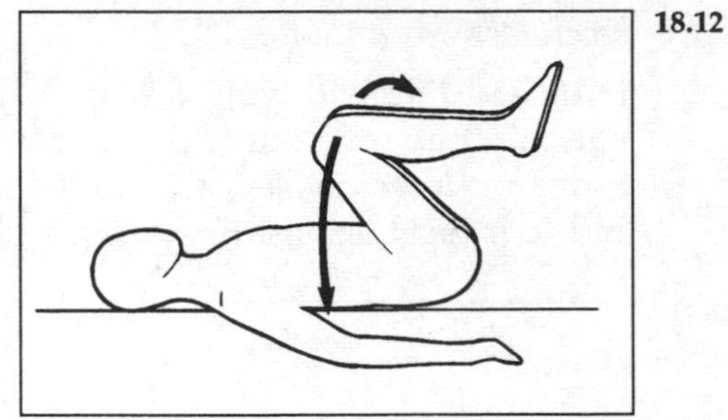

18.12

18.12 High knee rolling

18.13 Sitting on a chair with a back that reaches to the mid thoracic spine: turn your shoulders round to the right, place your right hand behind the chair and your left hand holding the side of the back, pull with your hands to help you turn round as far as you can. Repeat to the left. 3–4 times each way.

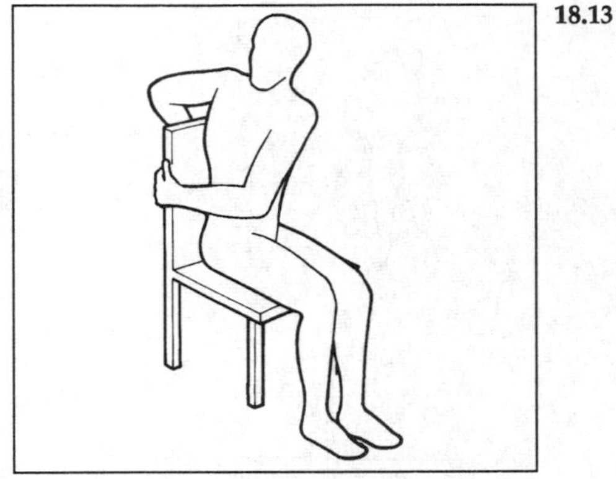

18.13

18.13 Passive rotation in sitting

18.14 Sitting on a stool:
For rotating the upper thoracic spine, leave your hands hanging by your side and turn slowly round to the left and then to the right as far as you can. Repeat 6 times.

For rotating the mid-thoracic area, repeat this with your elbows bent and hands touching your shoulders.

For rotating the lower thoracic spine, repeat the same movement with your arms stretched above your head (Comerford, 1993).

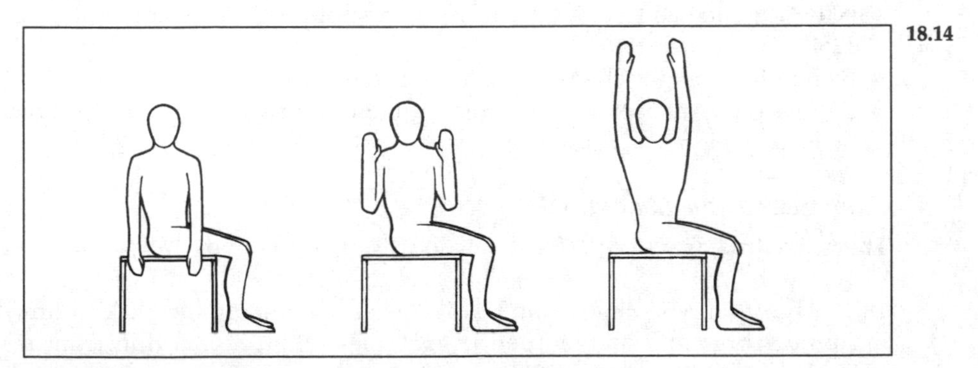

18.14

18.14 Rotation in sitting with change of arm position

Exercises for side flexion

18.15 Standing with your feet slightly apart, 10–15 cm away from a wall, lean back and rest your back flat against the wall. Bend to the left stretching your arm down one leg as far as it will go, keeping the whole of your back and your head against the wall, give three little pushes to the left and then straighten up. Repeat three times to the left. Then repeat the sequence to the right three times (Comerford, 1993).

18.15

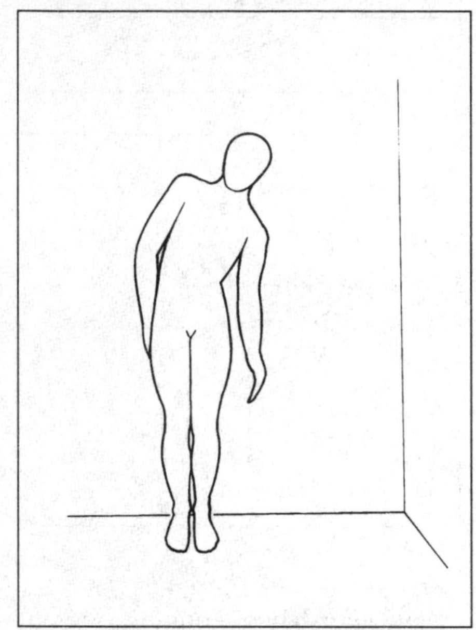

Repeat **18.15** with the right arm swinging over the head as you bend to the left. Repeat the opposite way *(not illustrated).*

Sitting on a chair, place both hands on your hips. Tilt the pelvis from side to side, rocking from one side to the other without disturbing the shoulder line *(not illustrated).*

18.15 Side flexion in standing – back against a wall

Strengthening exercises

Muscle strength can be increased in different ways, those that concern us here are:

- By static muscle work, a postural endurance hold in which anti-gravity muscles are contracted and held, first as an exercise, then as a 'red-dot' exercise and maintained while you are performing everyday activities such as cleaning your teeth or shopping (see Chapter 11, p. 125) (Comerford, 1993).
- By repetitive contractions in and out of a position.
- By resisted exercises, for example by using either gravity, one's own body, or weights as resistance.

Exercises for the abdominal muscles

There are three ways of performing a localised abdominal contraction:

18.16 Abdominal bracing, as on p. 194. Used for bracing the back in lifting procedures and as therapeutic exercises when recovering from a painful episode (Kennedy, 1980).

18.17 Abdominal hollowing. Crook lying, hollow or suck in your abdomen, allowing your ribs to 'flare'. *Do not* lift your chest. Do *not* tilt the pelvis back but allow the lumbar spine to flatten slightly. Hold for a count of 20. Relax. This exercise uses your **abdominal oblique muscles**. Practice it in lying, then in standing and use as a 'red-dot' exercise hundreds of times a day (Comerford, 1993).

18.16

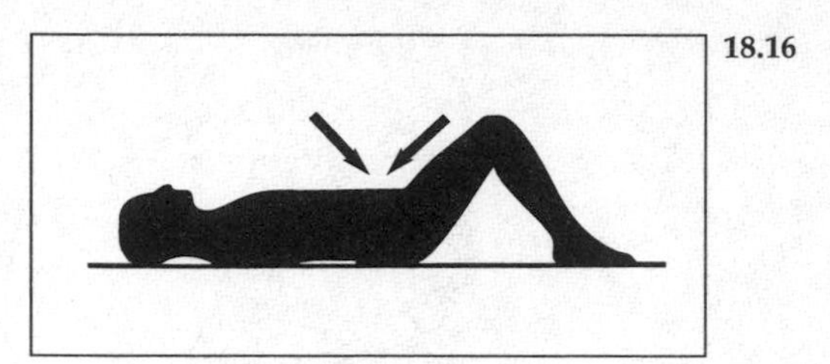

18.16 Abdominal bracing

18.17

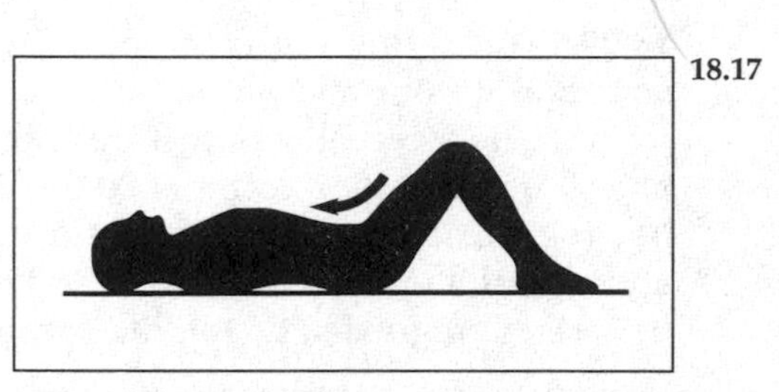

18.17 Abdominal hollowing

18.18 Pelvic tilting. Crook lying, pull your abdomen in until the lumbar spine is flat against the floor, hold for a count of 20 seconds while you go on breathing, then relax. The pelvis should tilt backwards as the lumbar spine presses against the floor. It might help to place your hands flat on the floor just under your waist so that you can feel the pressure as your spine pushes back. Repeat 5–6 times. This uses the **rectus abdominis** muscle.

18.18

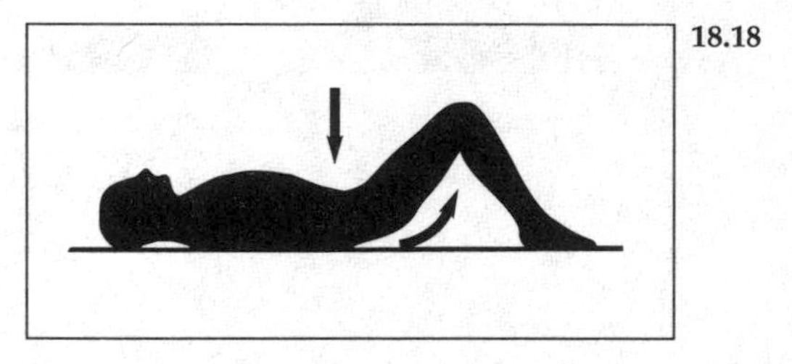

18.18 Pelvic tilting

18.19 Lying with the left knee bent and the right leg straight: tighten the abdominal muscles, keep them under control, tighten the right quadriceps muscles and slowly lift the right leg up and down 10 times. Lower and relax. Repeat with the other leg. Repeat 10 times on each side.

18.19

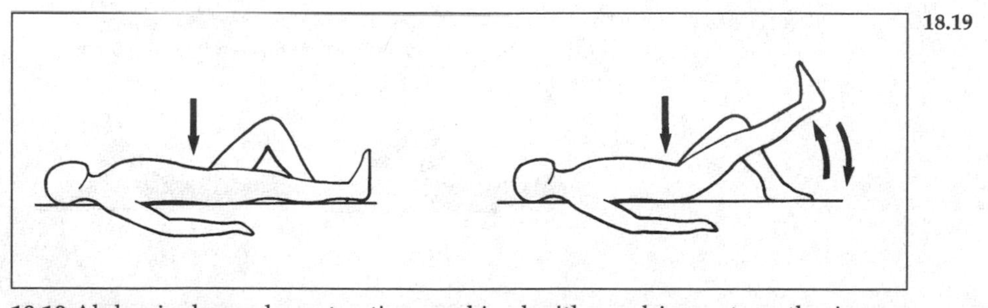

18.19 Abdominal muscle contraction combined with quadriceps strengthening

18.20

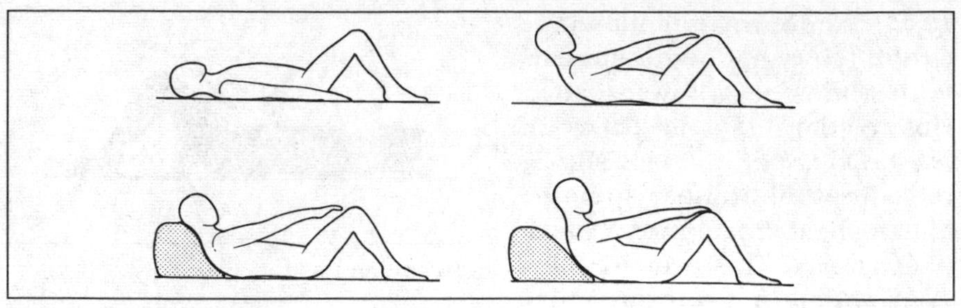

18.20 Abdominal curl-up

18.20 Crook lying flat or crook lying on a pillow (depending on the strength of your abdominal muscles), raise your head and shoulders from the floor reaching both arms towards your knees about half way up to a sit-up, hold for a count of 20 then lower. Repeat 5–10 times. This can be progressed to a sit-up, but be sure you curl your back up as you do so and uncurl it on the way down. Do not keep it straight. The exercise can be further progressed by folding your arms.

18.21

Crook lying...

...tighten your abdominal muscles, pressing your waist back on to the floor...

...hold your abdominal muscles tight while you pull both knees up...

NO!

...to your chest...

...hold your abdominal muscles tight while you lower your knees back to the floor. Relax. Repeat 3–10 times.

NO!

NO!

18.21 LOW abdominal contraction

18.22 Crook lying, pull both knees up towards your shoulders as high as you can without using your hands, lifting your buttocks off the ground. Lower back to crook lying. Repeat 5–10 times.

18.22

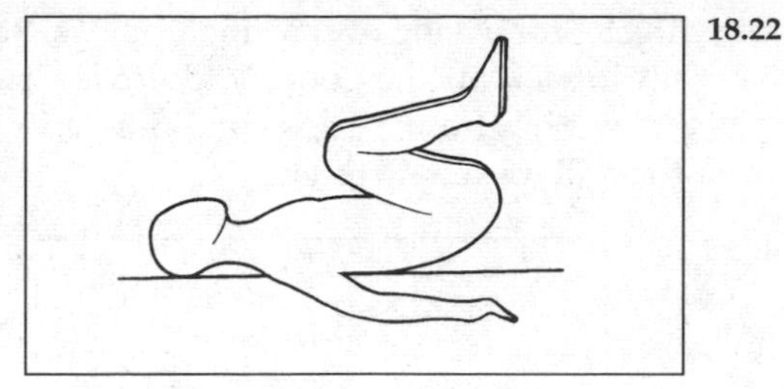

18.22 High abdominal contraction

18.23 Lying supine, pull your left knee up towards your right shoulder, place your right hand on the knee and push so that your hand is stopping the movement of your knee, hold for a count of 5, then let go slowly and relax. Repeat 3 times with each leg, or repeat alternately. The amount of resistance you give depends upon your ability, gradually increase it as you become stronger.

18.23

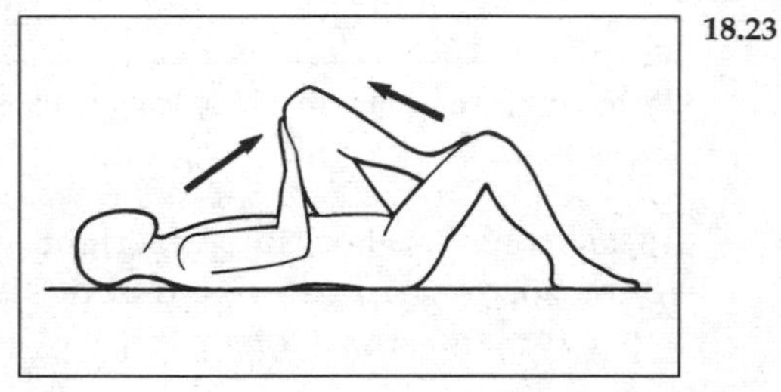

18.23 Contraction of the oblique abdominal muscles by resisting hip flexion

Exercises for the back extensor muscles

18.24 Prone lying with a pillow under your abdomen, raise your head and shoulders just up from the floor, not above the level of your hips, hold, then lower. Repeat 3–6 times.

18.24

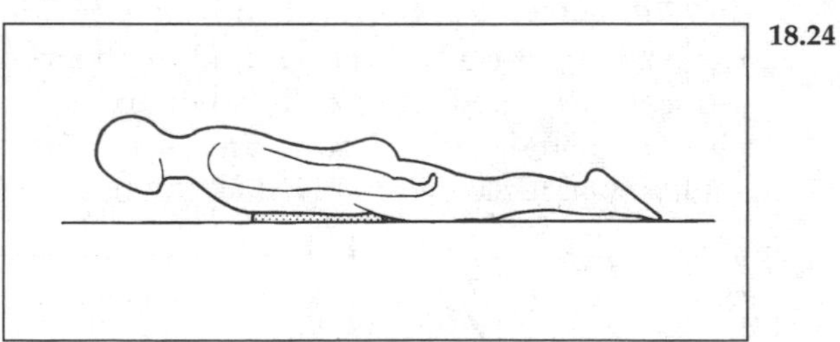

18.24 Gentle back extension

As above without the pillow (*not illustrated)*. If you are recovering from a back condition do not raise your shoulders above the horizontal.

18.25 Prone lying over a small pillow, keeping one leg stretched out straight, lift it back off the floor, hold, lower. Repeat with the other leg. If you are recovering from a back condition do not lift the leg higher than your buttocks. Repeat 5–10 times.

18.25

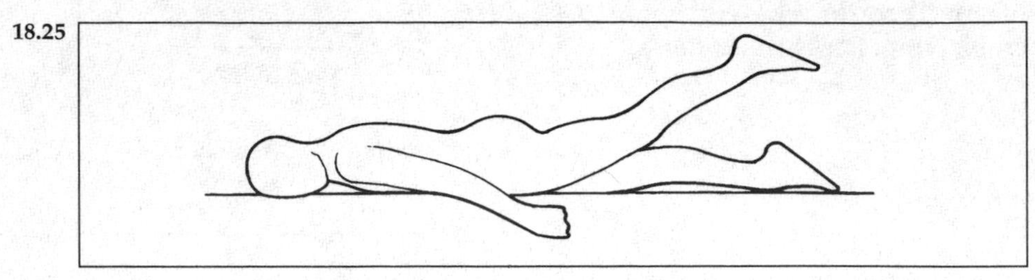

18.25 Hip extension with static back extensor muscle work

18.26 Prone kneeling, lift your right arm forwards and your left leg back to the horizontal, hollow your abdomen, hold and lower. Repeat with the other arm and leg 3–4 times.

18.26

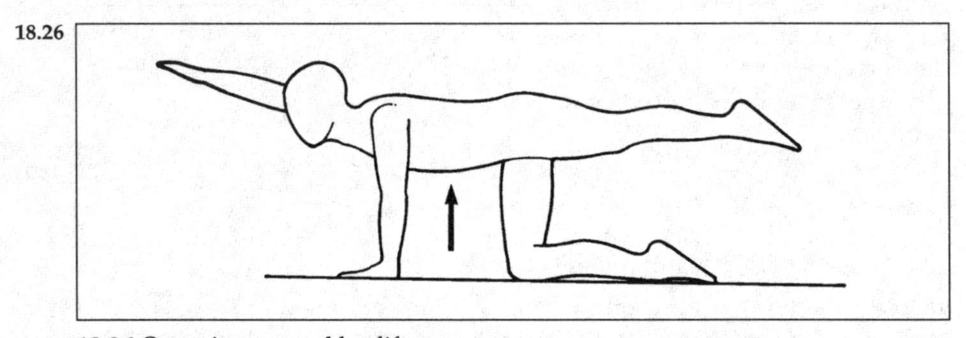

18.26 Opposite arm and leg lift

18.27 Prone lying with your hands by your side, lift your head and shoulders and both legs off the ground at the same time, trying to stretch or elongate your body as you do so, then lower. This is a very strong exercise and should not be done unless you are completely fit. Lift only as high as you feel comfortably able. Repeat 3–5 times.

18.27

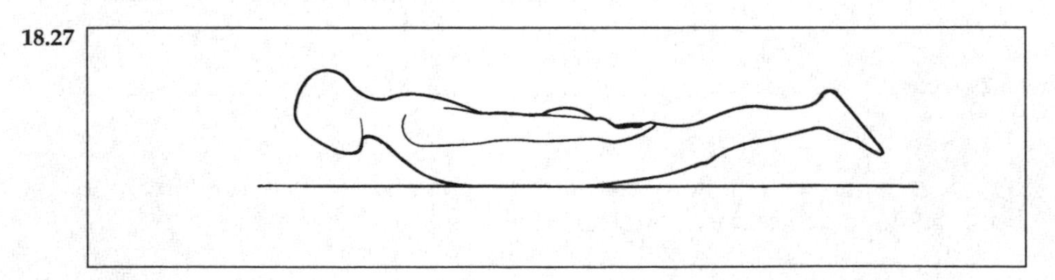

18.27 Strong back extension

Corrective exercises for a poking chin

18.28 Sitting on a stool with the whole of your back and head back resting against the wall, gently stretch the back of your head up the wall and the relax. Repeat 3–5 times. As you do this your chin should retract slightly but *do not* drop it towards your chest. When you have a good feel of this movement against the wall, do it as a postural correction in free sitting or standing (Comerford, 1993).

18.28

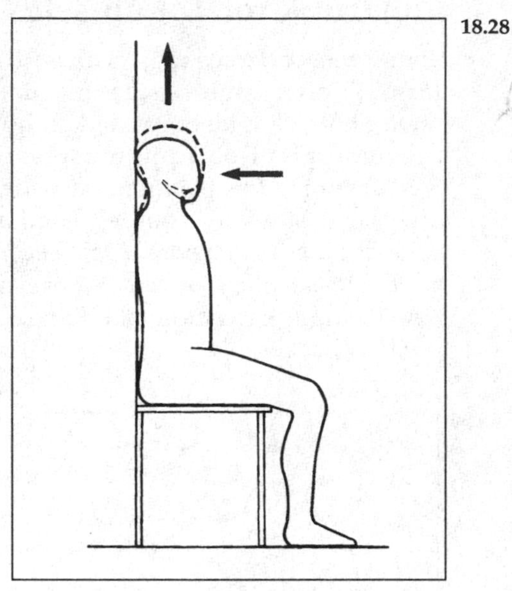

18.28 Head climbing up the wall – 'poking chin' correction

18.29 (from Gwendolen A Jull, *Headaches of Cervical Origin, Physical Therapy of the Cervical and Thoracic spine* (ed. Ruth Grant) Churchill Livingstone New York, 1988. With kind permission of author and publishers). Lie face downwards at the end of a firm bed with your chin hanging over the end into space.

Keeping your face parallel to the floor (do not tip your chin up), retract your chin, hold it retracted, then pull both shoulders back. Hold the position for a count of three. Relax your shoulders, then relax your chin. Repeat three times.

Do not perform this exercise if you are in pain. Seek the advice of a therapist first.

18.29

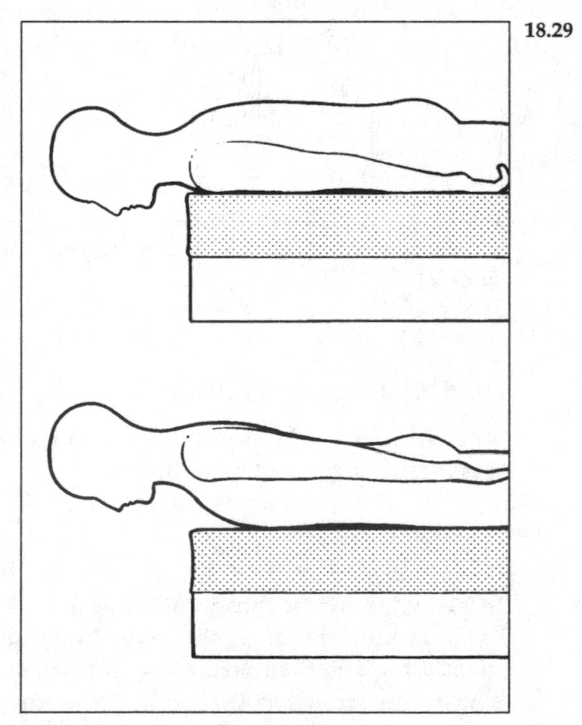

18.29 Chin retraction in lying

Stabilising exercise for abdominal, back extensor and trunk rotator muscles

Sitting well back on a table with both thighs fully supported.
18.30 1. Correct your posture maintaining a natural lordosis (not exagerrated), both shoulders relaxed; 2. hollow your abdomen by contracting the abdominal oblique muscles; 3. retract your chin; 4. sit tall. 5. Maintaining this position, lift your left knee from the table, 6. pushing down against it with your left hand and hold for a count of 20 seconds – *make sure that you do not tip onto one hip more than the other and that you do not twist your pelvis forwards on one side.* Relax. Correct again and repeat with the right knee and hand. Repeat 3–6 times (Comerford, 1993).

18.30

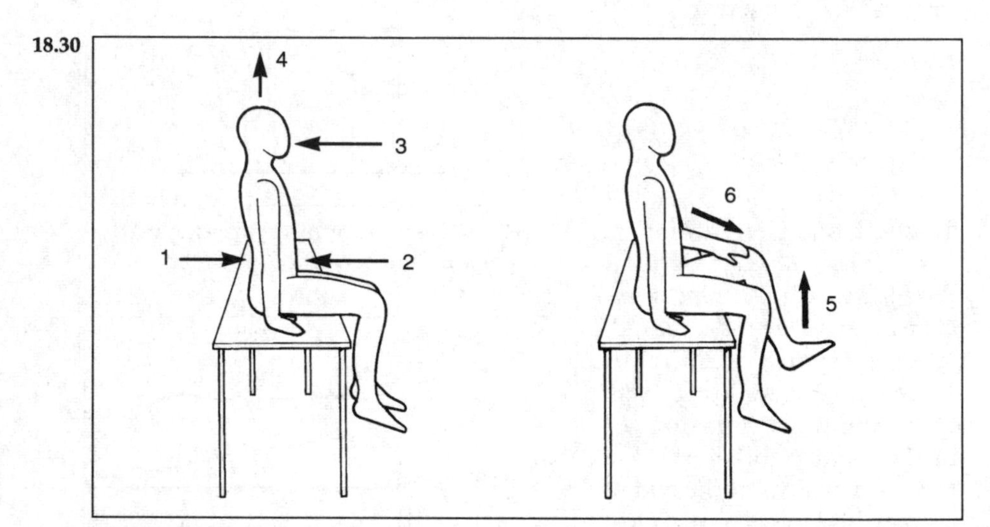

18.30 Stabilising exercise for abdominals, back extensors and trunk rotator muscles

Stretching exercises

Stretching should not be performed with a painful back unless specifically suggested by a therapist.

Hamstring stretching

18.31 Lying supine, straighten one leg as high as it will go, place your hands around the thigh above the knee and bend the knee. Pull the thigh *slightly* higher, then straighten and bend the knee slowly, feeling the hamstrings stretch at the back of the knee on each straightening movement of the leg. Repeat 5–10 times with each leg.

18.31

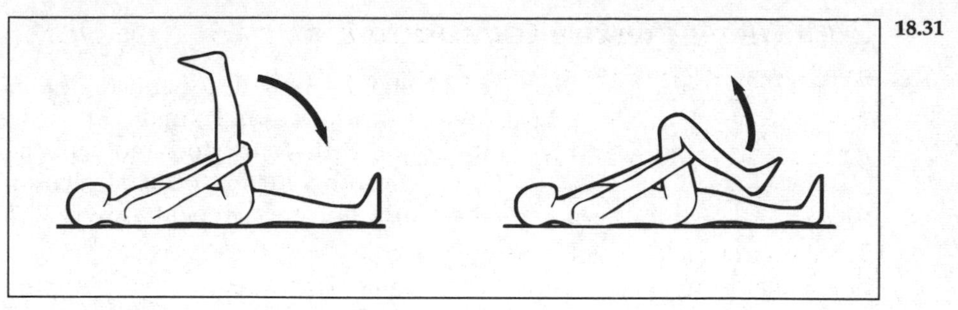

18.31 Hamstring muscle stretching

Two more advanced hamstring stretches are:

18.32

18.32 Sitting on a table, straighten one leg, hold it straight and then arch the lumbar spine. Hold for a count of 5, then slowly relax. Repeat with the other leg 3–5 times.

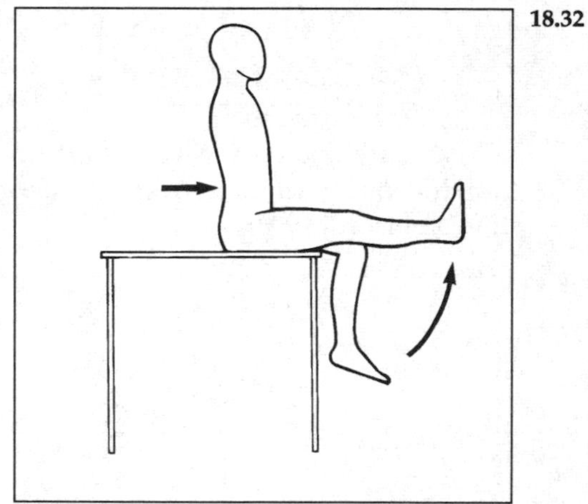

18.32 Hamstring stretch in sitting

18.33

18.33 Standing sideways on to a table, with the right foot on the floor, place the left leg flat along the edge of the table, arch the lumbar spine, hold and then relax. Repeat 3–5 times then change legs.

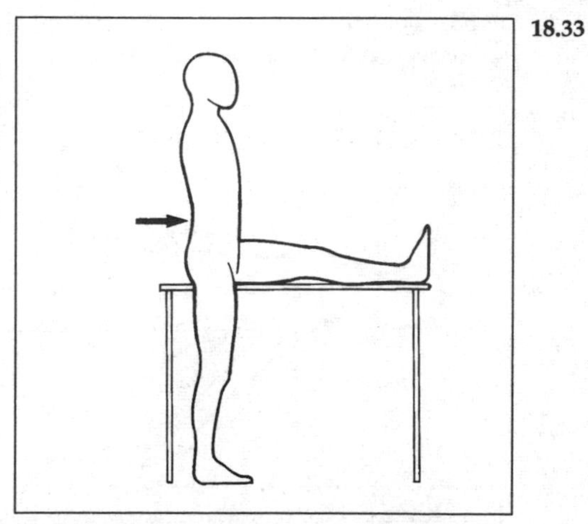

18.33 Hamstring stretch on a table

Quadriceps stretching

18.34

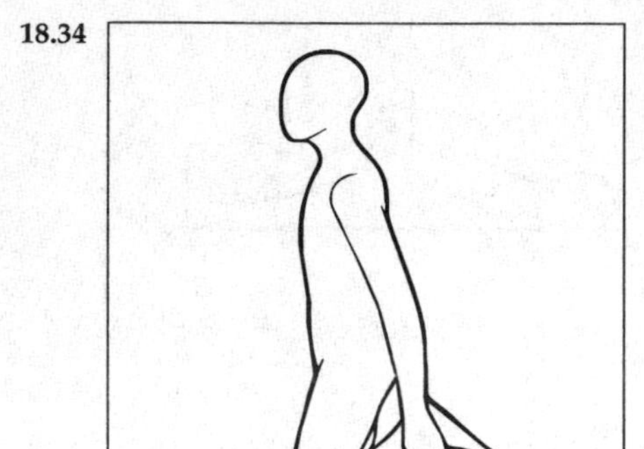

18.34 Stand on one leg, bend the other knee up with the foot behind you, grasp the ankle with your hand and pull the heel towards your buttocks, stretching the thigh muscles. Repeat slowly 2–3 times.

18.34 Quadriceps muscle stretching

There are different ways of performing this exercise: **18.35** is a precise quadriceps stretching movement, and **18.36** adds a trunk stabilisation to it (Comerford, 1993).

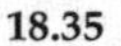

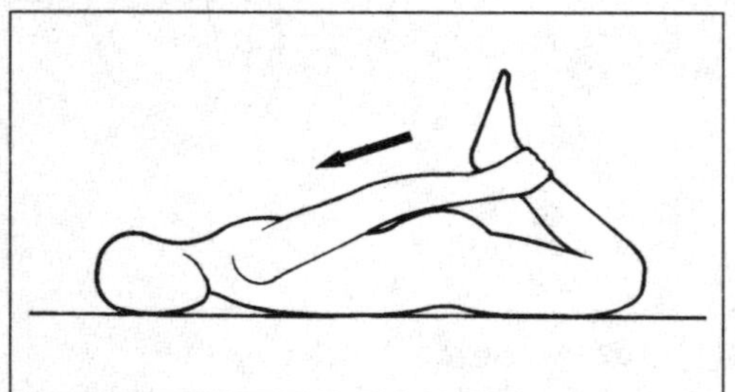

18.35 Quadriceps stretching by pulling the lower leg up towards the buttocks

18.35 Prone lying, bend the right knee with the heel trying to reach the buttocks, pull the leg up further either by gripping the ankle with your right hand or by hooking a towel or belt round the ankle. Hold for a count of 3–5. Repeat 3–5 times with each leg.

18.36

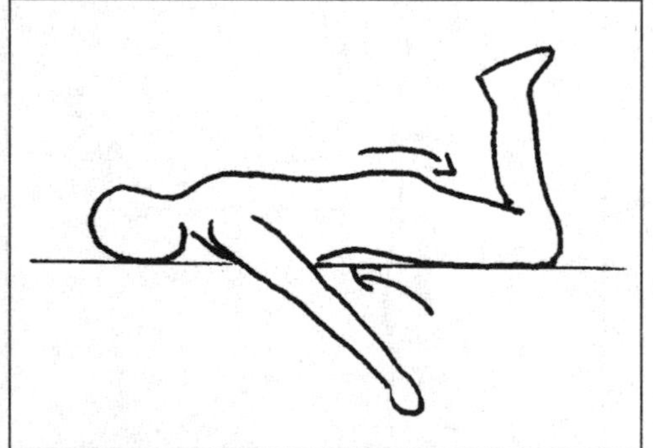

18.36 Knee bending, stabilising the pelvic tilt

18.36 Prone lying, tighten the buttocks and hollow the abdomen, tilting the pelvis back; hold this while you bend your knee as far as possible without releasing the pelvis. Hold for a count of 10. Lower thw leg and relax. Repeat 5 times.

Hip and knee stretching

18.37 and **18.38** are gentle hip and knee stretches for older joints.

18.37 Stand with one leg behind you, resting the toe on the ground. Keep your body upright and your pelvis still, and *do not* lean forwards or rotate the pelvis. Straighten the knee of the back leg firmly, tighten the thigh and stretch the front of the hip. Then relax, leaving the toe where it is. Repeat 5–10 times.

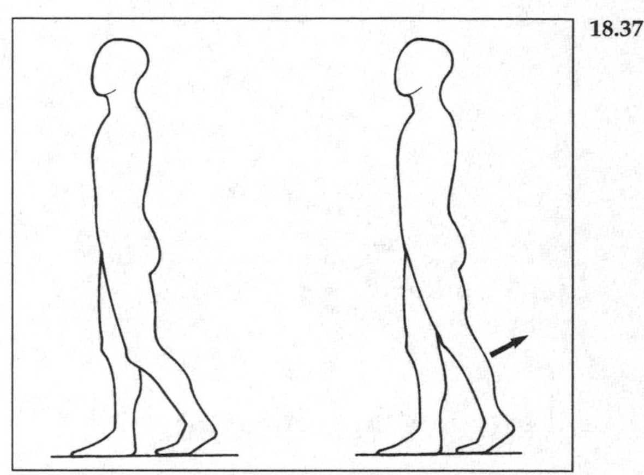

18.37 Gentle hip and knee joint extension

18.38 Lying supine, bend one knee up towards your chest, hold it with both hands and pull it as high as you can while pressing the straight leg onto the ground so that you are pulling in one direction and stretching in the other. Give 3–4 pulls with each leg.

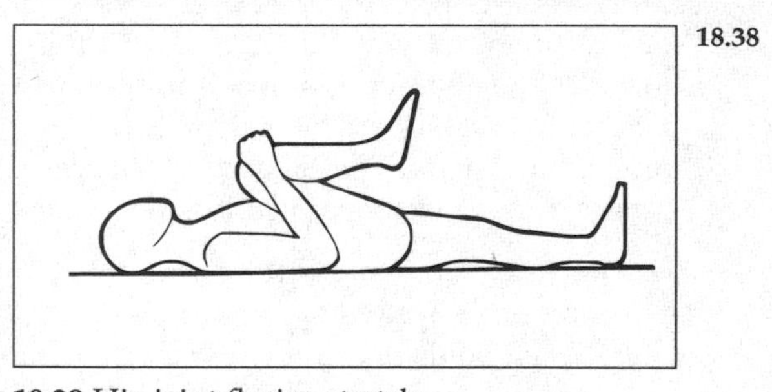

18.38 Hip joint flexion stretch

18.39 Stand in the forward lunge position with the front knee bent and the back knee straight. Bend the front knee further, lowering your hips and stretching the front of the hip joint. Hold for a count of 20 or do 6–10 slow stretches.

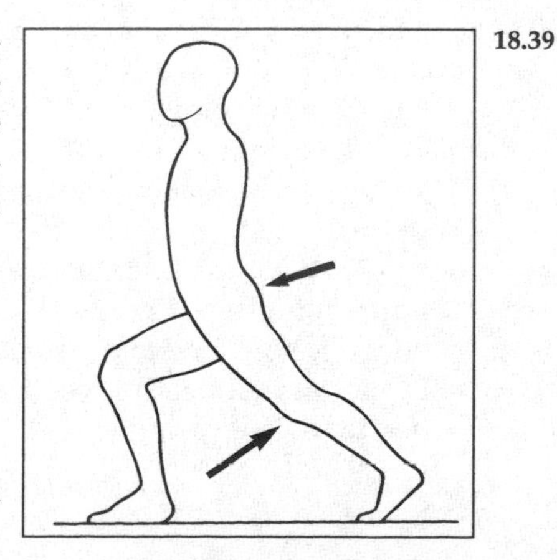

18.39 Stronger hip joint extension stretch (stretching the hip flexor muscles)

18.40

18.40 Hip abduction (sideways) stretch

18.40 Stand on one leg and lift the other leg sideways as high as you can and then lower. Make sure you remain upright and that you do not lean the other way as you lift the leg. Repeat 5–10 times with each leg.

Exercises for endurance

Endurance (a measure of fitness) is the ability to work for prolonged periods of time and the ability to resist fatigue (Kisner and Colby, 1988). It includes the endurance of local musculature and that of the body systems. Both are necessary for the performance of repeated tasks, such as walking or climbing stairs. Typical endurance sports are swimming, walking, running, skipping, cycling (including the static bike) and aerobics.

- The exercise or activity should be performed for between 15–45 minutes, 3–5 days a week, but adequate rest periods are essential between bouts of training (Kisner and Colby, 1988).
- A good warm-up before starting is essential. This should include stretching and slow gentle movements, gradually increasing the rate and effort you are making until ready for action.
- Good equipment is important, for example, good shoes or the right length of skipping rope.
- The environment of your activity is also important, if you are lucky enough to be able to choose. Running on soft ground in parkland or countryside is preferable to running on hard pavements in town.
- Avoid strain or overuse of muscles which can occur if you do too much too often. Record the exercise you do, keeping an account of how far, how long and how hard you have worked.
- Do not attempt endurance training unless you are fit; consult a doctor if you are in any doubt.

Classes for rehabilitation and maintaining fitness

Keep fit: keep fit classes of all kinds operate throughout the country offering different forms of training. They vary in standard and regime provided. You need to investigate and choose one that suits your particular requirements. There are many special classes for the older person.

Yoga: there are many misconceptions about Yoga; it is imagined to be a form of dreamy mysticism which somehow also involves tying the body into knots. In fact, Yoga is about achieving physical and mental health in a very practical way. Physically it involves a series of stretching actions which increase the mobility of the body by continually taking the joints and tissues into their full range in careful, unstressed movements. Mentally, the poses themselves become meditative through the quiet focusing of the mind on the activity of the body. By extending one's consciousness into these cells of the body which are habitually unaware, Yoga unites mind and body. The word Yoga means yoke or union.

Aerobics: aerobics develops endurance and strength. The teacher should be fully-qualified and you should ensure that you are fit to participate in the classes.

Exercises to avoid

There are three exercises that are unacceptable, two for the back and one for the neck.

- Lying supine, do not lift both legs together at the same time.
- Lying supine, do not do sit-ups with straight legs.
  (These two exercises put a considerable strain upon the lumbar spine as they cause a mechanical conflict with musculature. They should only be performed under expert training and supervision).
- Neck-circling exercise. This exercise, which is often used in exercise classes, screws the cervical spine round in a complicated range of combined movements; it stresses the joints quite unproductively and provides no beneficial effect.

REFERENCES

Adams, M.A. and Hutton, W.C. (1983). The effect of posture on the fluid content of lumbar intervertebral discs, *Spine*, **8**(6).

Baum, G. (1991). *Aquarobics*, Arrow Books.

Comerford, M. (1993)(personal communication).

Jull, G. (1988). Headaches of cervical origin, *Physical Therapy of the Cervical and Thoracic Spine* (Grant, R., ed.), Churchill Livingstone, New York.

Kennedy, B. (1980). An Australian programme for management of back problems, *Physiotherapy*, **66**(4), 108–111.

Kisner, C. and Colby, L.A. (1988). *Therapeutic Exercises. Foundations and Techniques*, F.A. Davis, Philadelphia.

McIntosh, P.C. (1979). Sport in society, *Sports Medicine* (Williams, J.G.P. and Sperryn, P.N., eds.), 2nd ed., Edward Arnold, London.
McKenzie, R. (1981). *The Lumbar Spine, Mechanical Diagnosis and Therapy*, Spinal Publications.
Muir Gray, J.A. (1987). Exercise and ageing, *Exercise, Benefits, Limits and Adaptations* (Macleod, D., Maughan, R., Nimmo, M., Reilly, T. and Williams, C., eds.), E. & F.N. Spon, New York.
Peterson, L. and Renstrom, P. (1992). *Sports Injuries*, Martin Dunitz.
Radin, E.L. and Paul I.L. (1972). A consolidated concept of joint lubrication, *J. Bone Joint Surg.*, **54A**(3).
Stubbs, D.A. (1982). Back problems in work and leisure, *Physiotherapy*, **68**(6).
Thomason, H. (1979). Joints, *Sports Medicine*, (Williams, J.G.P. and Sperryn P.N., eds.), 2nd ed., Edward Arnold, London.
Twomey, L. (1989). Physical activity and ageing bones, *Patient Management 'Focus'*, **August**, 27–34.
Twomey, L. (1992) (personal communication).
Twomey, L.T. and Taylor, J.R. (1987). Lumbar posture, movements and mechanics, *Physical Therapy of the Low Back* (Twomey, L.T. and Taylor, J.R., eds.), Churchill Livingstone, USA.
Twomey, L.T. and Taylor, J.R. (1991). Age-related changes of the lumbar spine and spinal rehabilitation. Reprinted from the *CRC Critical Reviews in Physical and Rehabilitation Medicine*, **2**(3), 153–169.
Twomey, L.T., Taylor, J.R. and Oliver, M.J. (1988). Sustained flexion loading, rapid extension loading of the lumbar spine, and the physical therapy of related injuries, *Physiotherapy Practice*, **4**, 129–137.
Waddell. G. (1989). A new clinical model for the treatment of back pain, *Back Pain: New Approaches for Rehabilitation and Education* (Martin, R. and Jenner, J.R., eds.), Manchester University Press.

19. Treatments available

The aim of this book has been to teach the reader to administer his/her own back care and develop a positive approach to pain. All too often the relief of pain requires help from other sources; these include medication, manipulative therapies, sensory modulation in the form of transcutaneous electrical nerve stimulation or acupuncture, or other forms of electrotherapy. Each of these will be discussed briefly below.

Medication

The benefit from and use of any medication is entirely dependent upon the cause and severity of the pain. Drugs can be used to affect pain at a wide range of sites along the sensory pathways, ranging from action against the pathological process producing pain to modulation of the cerebral response at the emotional level (Baxter, 1988). Only those more commonly used in the treatment of back pain are discussed here.

Non-narcotic analgesics and anti-inflammatory drugs

Non-narcotic analgesics, including aspirin, paracetamol and the huge group of non steroidal anti-inflammatory drugs (NSAIDs), constitute a mixed group of compounds differing in chemical structure but sharing certain pharmaceutical and therapeutic actions (Melzack and Wall, 1991).

These drugs act on the injured tissue itself, and are thus described as peripherally-acting compounds. Many of these peripherally-acting analgesics possess analgesic, antipyretic and anti-inflammatory properties, except for paracetamol whose anti-inflammatory activity is weak (Sunshine, 1989).

Mechanical pain, triggered by non-inflammatory reaction, does not respond to anti-inflammatory medication (Melzack and Wall, 1991). However, in most traumatically induced episodes there is an inflammatory element and drugs can be of value in reducing pain to a tolerable level, to alleviate muscle spasm and assist sleep. Sleep is both psychologically and physiologically important for the process of healing and nourishment of tissues.

Tranquillisers and muscle relaxants

Tranquillisers and muscle relaxants have some value in allaying anxiety or aiding sleep but Baxter (1988) feels their role is dubious, especially with the possible hazard of addiction. Diazepam, however, does have useful muscle relaxant properties and for this reason can be of value in cases of extreme protective spasm (ibid).

Steroids

Steroids are potent reducers of tissue swelling and are used either locally in injection form, to reduce swelling in acute conditions, or by medication in conditions such as rheumatoid arthritis. Their long term use can, however, lead to osteoporotic changes in bone.

Physiotherapy

Physiotherapy is a health care profession which emphasises the use of physical approaches in the prevention and treatment of disease and disability (CSP, 1991).

Physiotherapy has changed dynamically since the late 1960s. Prior to that there was minimal specialisation, and in the musculoskeletal field, physiotherapy consisted of electrotherapy, heat, massage and exercises. Cyriax was the only advocate of any manipulative procedure.

In the 1960s Grieve (1981) and Maitland (1991 and 1992) pioneered the way into a new approach of musculoskeletal assessment and treatment. As always, new ideas stimulate further investigation. New techniques relating to vertebral mobilisation (for example, Grant, 1988; Edwards, 1992) and soft tissue treatments (for example, Palastanga, 1991; Weintraube, 1991) are constantly developing. Latterly, neural tissue is being looked at in completely new ways (Elvey *et al.*, 1986; Elvey, 1991; Butler 1991) as is muscle funcion and imbalance (Kendall and McCleary, 1983; Sahrmann, 1987; Richardson *et al.*, 1992).

Before 1977 treatment could only be carried out with medical diagnosis and referral by a doctor. A health circular issued by the DHSS in 1977 removed this requirement (Bithell, 1992), allowing Chartered Physiotherapists to make their own assessment and treatment decisions. This assessment takes into account: '*...the patients' current psychological, cultural and social factors, and is based on an assessment of movement and function. The aim is to identify and diagnose the specific components of movement and function responsible for the patients' physical problems*' (CSP, 1991).

The physiotherapist carefully notes the story of the patient's injury or problem, together with any other pains or symptoms which may be present, including the past history of previous ailments. There follows a meticulous objective examination which includes active body movements, passive movements of joints, evaluation of the accessory joint movements (those which cannot be performed actively), palpation of all relevant soft tissue, muscle testing, and neurological examination. In this examination the physiotherapist is looking for any signs which match up with the patient's symptoms.

The final result should be a diagnosis of malfunction in specific areas or tissues of the body which the physiotherapist will then treat by means of mobilisation of the joints and/or soft tissue, manipulation if necessary, soft tissue stretching, traction, muscular re-education, postural correction and advice, exercises and any electrical treatment deemed applicable. Treatment is always concluded with a home programme of exercises to reinforce progress and to try to prevent further recurrence.

For two or three years after qualifying, physiotherapists usually work in general hospitals gaining experience in all fields. They then choose one of the following specialities for postgraduate training: paediatrics, respiratory care, care of the elderly, neurology, orthopaedics or sports injuries and musculoskeletal conditions. They may continue to work in the National Health Service or in private practice.

If you require treatment for a back condition, any physiotherapist you consult should be a member of the Chartered Society of Physiotherapy (MCSP), or even better, one who has special interests in the treatment of spinal and other joint disorders.

Other manipulative therapies

Osteopathy

Osteopathy started in the USA in 1892. Since then it has flourished both in the USA, UK and parts of Europe (Belshaw, 1987). It is the science of human mechanics, a system of diagnosis and manual treatment which places its main emphasis on the structural and mechanical problems of the body.

Osteopaths are concerned with the biomechanics of the body and the maintenance of proper mechanical function. Osteopathy can ensure that the musculoskeletal system is functioning to its optimum potential. It can do for the body's framework what a service will do for a car – identify existing and potential problems and ensure that all parts are in good working order (Munro and Forster, 1992).

Treatment uses predominantly gentle manual methods of articulatory techniques and soft tissue stretching, and a diagnostic procedure similar to a conventional medical examination but with particular attention to detailed assessment of the patient's musculoskeletal system. Osteopaths treat tension headaches, neck and shoulder pain, joint strains in all parts of the body, pains and discomfort associated with pregnancy and sports injuries (Munro and Forster, 1992).

Registered osteopaths are members of the General Council and Register of Osteopaths and have MRO after their name.

Chiropractic

Chiropractors specialise in diagnosing and treating disorders of the spine, joints and muscles. The term is derived form the Greek words *chiero* (hands) and *praktos* (to use), and means treatment by hand or manipulation. Chiropractors will take a thorough case history and carry out a full neurological and orthopaedic examination. They may also take X-rays to check for any abnormalities or conditions which will show if another form of treatment would be more appropriate. The chiropractor then carries out a detailed analysis of how the individual bones, joints and muscles move, in order to identify the specific problem area (Bennett, 1992).

Treatment consists of gently unlocking the stiff joints with skilled manipulations, known as adjustment. Quick, comfortable adjustments are used with just the right amount of pressure to restore proper function and mobility to joints. Chiropractors treat all musculoskeletal pain (Bennett, 1992).

The British Chiropractic Association is the representative body for the profession and maintains a register of fully qualified chiropractors who should have BCA after their name.

Sensory modulation of pain

Transcutaneous electrical nerve stimulation (TENS)

Transcutaneous electrical nerve stimulation is a pulsed electrical current which is used for pain relief. It is based on the gate control theory (p. 91). TENS stimulates the large, fast-conducting nerve fibres which override the smaller, slower, afferent fibres conducting noxious stimuli thus closing the gate of pain perception (Lewith, 1984; Frampton, 1988). The apparatus consists of a small box about 8cm square which can be carried around in a pocket, and from which two or four leads carry the current to rubber electrodes placed on the skin. It is used for long-standing severe pain, chronic pain, post-herpetic neuralgia, phantom limb pain and during labour (Thomson *et al.*, 1991).

Acupuncture

Acupuncture is an old and well-tried treatment of pain used for hundreds of years in China. It was originally treated suspiciously by Western medicine but is now being used more and more in clinical situations, with medical referrals to acupuncturists. Special needles are inserted at strategic places and vibrated to produce a sensory input; electrical currents are sometimes passed through the needles as added stimulation.The effect is again based on the gate control theory and recent investigation by Melzack found that the precise factor is the intense degree of stimulation, the site of the stimulation being less important than the output (Melzack, 1989).

Other electrical modalities

Ultrasound

Ultrasound is the production of high-frequency mechanical waves above the audible range of sound, generated by a piezo-electric or quartz crystal called a transducer. The crystal is housed in a small torch-like casing or even a smaller thick pencil shaped instrument. The area to be treated is creamed and the instrument head is moved slowly over it, maintaining contact throughout. It can also be used in a water bath.

The vibration of the current oscillates the particles in the fluid content of the tissue cells, stimulating the release of chemical mediators which accelerates the healing process (Kitchen and Partridge, 1990).

Ultrasound is used to treat many conditions from open wounds, such as leg ulcers, to sprains and sports injuries, traumatic bruising, post-operative scarring and muscle spasm – in fact wherever there is local tenderness, swelling and inflammation. It will not help mechanical pain. Ultrasound is mostly without sensation but warmth can be felt, depending upon the type of current used.

Interferential

Interferential is an electrical stimulation using two medium-frequency currents to produce a low-frequency effect within the body. It is applied with two or four pads which can be of the suction type or flat pads encased in wet foam rubber. By varying the frequency of the current it is possible to treat all types of muscle and nervous tissue – motor, sensory, sympathetic and parasympathetic. It is used for the treatment of pain, swelling, inflammation, muscular re-education and for conditions which require an increase of circulation (Major, 1992).

Laser

'Laser' is an acronym for Light Amplification by Stimulated Emission of Radiation. Specific substances are stimulated electrically to emit radiations which produce greater energy levels. The beam of light emitted is narrow. Laser therapy is used for tissue repair, wound healing and pain relief. The effects spread from one cell to another and therefore to surrounding tissue (Thomson *et al.*, 1991).

Short wave diathermy (SWD) or pulsed electromagnetic energy (PEME)

Short wave diathermy or pulsed electromagnetic energy is an oscillating electromagnetic field which affects the molecules in the tissues. Heat is generated in unpulsed SWD and it is used to treat both deep and superficial tissue. It is nowadays used more frequently in its pulsed form for pain relief in acute soft tissue lesions, obtaining a marked reduction in local swelling; it is also used in wound healing (ibid).

Investigative procedures

Radiography or X-ray

X-rays are a non-invasive tool in which a beam of radiation is passed through the body providing pictures which show shadows of the bones, leaving us to guess the condition of the more important soft tissues (Porter, 1986; Mourad, 1991). They show fractures, degenerative changes, disc narrowing, osteophytes, Schmorl's nodes, bony anomalies such as spondylolisthesis, and bony diseases; oblique views can show the sizes of the intervertebral foramina.

Myelography or radiculography

Myelography is contrast radiography. It has now been replaced by the CT scan, but when this is unavailable myelography is still used.

A water-soluble contrast medium, metrizamide, is used and injected into the spinal canal at the disc space in order to show up any abnormalities present. X-rays are then taken of the spine. The metrizamide is absorbed into the blood stream with few complications. Oil-based contrast media have far greater side effects such as nausea, vomiting, headaches, arachnoiditis and disorientation (Kirkaldy-Willis and Tchang, 1988).

Myelograms show disc herniation within the confines of the spinal canal and anterior or anterolateral defects within the vertebral column but they never demonstrate disc herniation in the lateral nerve canal. Tumour, neurofibromas and extradural abscesses are clearly shown (ibid).

Discography

Discography involves injecting a contrast medium into the disc in order to fill the area of the nucleus. The amount of injection material required to fill the nucleus depends on the state of the disc. The grossly degenerate disc has virtually no limit to the volume that can be injected (Porter, 1986). The discs are then X-rayed. The radiological appearances of normal and degenerate discs are quite characteristic. The outline of the degenerate nucleus is irregular and the 'tissue sequestrum' can be identified (ibid). Patients may experience pain during discography.

Facet arthrography

Facet arthrography is a similar technique for confirming or discounting the Z joint as a source of trouble; local anaesthetic is injected into the suspect joint or joints in order to ascertain the effect on the pain.

Radioisotope bone scan

Radioisotope bone scans record the concentration of radioactivity in the bone after the injection of radioactive technetium; they are useful for locating cancer, infection and inflammation (Eisenstein, 1992).

Computerised tomography (CT) scan

Computerised tomography is a non-invasive technique now widely used to diagnose lesions in the spine. With the use of high-resolution scanning, cross-sectional views of the of the spine are made; it is now possible to demonstrate soft tissue shadows and the nature of the soft tissue can be assessed with reasonable accuracy. By rotating the patient on the examination table it is possible to study the effect of movement upon the Z joints and the lateral canals (Kirkaldy-Willis and Tchang, 1988; Eisenstein, 1992).

Magnetic resonance imaging (MRI)

MRI is another non-invasive procedure in which very high magnetic forces are sent through the body to alter the alignment of hydrogen ions in the nuclei of cells. When irradiation stops, the nuclear atoms return to their original position, emitting the absorbed energy as signals that are stored by computer and projected as images (Mourad, 1991). It has proved to be a useful adjunct to the CT scan. It provides markedly improved soft tissue contrast resolution of discs and neural elements, as well as the capability of imaging in multiple planes. The improved soft tissue resolution shows clear differentiation between structures such as disc material, neural elements, intraspinal haematoma and spinal tumours (Heithoff, 1988).

Electromyography

Routine nerve conduction studies often appear normal in patients with nerve root lesions. However, they help to exclude other conditions such as neuropathy which may confuse diagnosis. Electromyography, an electrical test, shows fibrillation potentials and motor unit changes in denervated muscle; the distribution of abnormalities may help to localise the lesion to a particular root. The EMG is negative in patients whose symptoms are due to irritation of the dorsal roots (Kirkaldy-Willis and Tchang, 1988).

Surgery

As a result of these investigations it might be found necessary to operate on the spine. The types of surgical procedures vary from removal of part of the disc to spinal fusions (Eisenstein, 1992). Descriptions of these operations are beyond the scope of this book and it is hoped that with back care followed religiously this step need never be taken.

REFERENCES

Baxter, R. (1988). Drug control of pain, *Pain. Management and Control in Physiotherapy* (Wells, P., Frampton, V. and Bowsher, D., eds.), Heinemann Medical Books.

Belshaw, C. (1987). *Osteopathy. Is it for you?* Element Books Ltd.

Bennet, M. (1992). *Chiropractic. What it is and How Does it Work?* British Chiropractic Association.

Bithell, C. (1992). The Olive Sands memorial lecture: clinical diagnosis, *In Touch. The Journal of the OCPPP*, **64**, 31–34.

Butler, D. (1991). *Mobilisation of the Nervous System*, Churchill Livingstone.

Chartered Society of Physiotherapy (1991). *Definition of Physiotherapy*, Curriculum of Study.

Edwards, B.C. (1992). *Manual of Combined Movements*, Churchill Livingstone.

Eisenstein, S. (1992). Surgery for spinal disorders, *Cash's Textbook of Orthopaedics and Rheumatology for Physiotherapists*, Mosby Year Book Europe.

Elvey, R.L., Quinter, J. and Thomas, A. (1986). A clinical study of RSI, *Australian Family Physician*, **15** (2), 10, 1314–1322.

Elvey, R.L. (1991). The investigation of arm pain, *Modern Manual Therapy* (Grieve, G.G., ed.) Churchill Livingstone, 530–535.

Frampton, V. (1988). Transcutaneous electrical nerve stimulation and chronic pain, *Pain. Management and Control in Physiotherapy*, (Wells, P., Frampton, V. and Bowsher, D., eds.), Heinemann Medical Books.

Grant, R. (1988). Dizziness testing and manipulation of the cervical spine, *Physical Therapy of the Cervical and Thoracic Spine* (Grant, R., ed.), Churchill Livingstone.

Grieve, G.G. (1981). *Common Vertebral Joint Problems*, Churchill Livingstone, 2nd ed., Churchill Livingstone.

Heithoff, K.B. (1988). *Magnetic Resonance Imaging of the Lumbar Spine, Managing Low Back Pain* (Kirkaldy-Willis, W.H., ed), 2nd ed., Churchill Livingstone.

Kendall, F.P. and McCleary, F.K. (1983). *Muscle: Testing and Function* ed 3. Waverly Press, USA.

Kirkaldy-Willis, W.H. and Tchang, S. (1988). Diagnostic techniques, *Managing Low Back Pain* (Kirkaldy-Willis, W.H., ed), 2nd ed., Churchill Livingstone.

Kitchen, S.S. and Partridge, C.J. (1990). A review of therapeutic ultrasound, *Physiotherapy*, **76**(10).

Lewith, G.T. (1984). Transcutaneous electrical nerve stimulation for pain relief, *The World of Medicine*, 15 January.

Maitland, G.D. (1991). *Vertebral Manipulation*, 6th ed., Butterworths.

Maitland, G.D. (1992). *Peripheral Manipulation*, 3rd ed., Butterworths.

Melzack, R. (1989). Folk medicine and the sensory modulation of pain, *Textbook of Pain* (Wall, P.D. and Melzack, R., eds.), 2nd ed., Churchill Livingstone.

Melzack, R. and Wall, P.D. (1991). *The Challenge of Pain*, Penguin Books.

Major, K. (1992). Principles of treatment following joint examination and assessment, *Cash's Textbook of Orthopaedics and Rheumatology for Physiotherapists* (Tidswell, M.E., ed.), Mosby Year Book Europe.

Mourad, L.A. (1991). *Orthopedic Disorders*, Mosby Year Book.
Munro and Forster public relations (1992). *Osteopathy – The Facts*, The General Council and Register of Osteopaths.
Palastanga, N. (1991). Connective tissue massage, *Modern Manual Therapy* (Grieve, G.G., ed.), 827–833, Churchill Livingstone.
Porter, R.W. (1986). *Management of Back Pain*, Churchill Livingstone.
Richardson, C., Jull, G., Toppenberg, R. and Comerford, M. (1992). Techniques for active lumbar stabilisation for spinal protection: A pilot study. *Australian Physiotherapy*, **38** (2).
Sahrmann, S. (1987). Posture and muscle imbalance, *Postgraduate advances in Physical Therapy* I-VIII. A comprehensive Independent learning office study course, Washington University School of Medicine.
Sunshine, A. and Olson, N. (1989). Non-narcotic analgesics, *Textbook of Pain*, (Wall, P.D. and Melzack, R., eds.), Churchill Livingstone.
Thomson, A., Skinner, A. and Piercy, J. (1991). T*idy's Physiotherapy*, 12th ed., Butterworths.
Weintraube, A. (1991). soft tissue mobilisation, *Modern Manual Therapy* (Grieve, G.G., ed.), 750–755 , Churchill Livingstone.

20. Conclusion

Whatever the cause, back pain demands attention. Pain that says, 'I don't like this, do something to relieve it' or pain that says, 'Oh, that hurts, but it feels good, just stretch it a bit more' are the two main guidelines to your response. Remember that back pain is usually a disturbance of function of the joint or the soft tissue caused by a mechanical or chemical irritation or a combination of both. The origin of the disturbance will lie in daily abuse, or lack of use, or trauma (untraceable or recognisable) or an inflammatory reaction, or a combination of them all.

Ignoring pain may appear heroic, but it is doubly unproductive: first, if abuse is present you are allowing it to continue without listening to the body's warning; second, you are not analysing the situation with the aim of avoiding any repetition or working towards a cure. Pain must be acknowledged, analysed and a decision taken on the best action:

- Is the pain one of stiffness and limitation of movement and therefore one to be worked? Providing your approach takes the form of controlled, careful stretches, followed by mobilising exercises, the pain should lessen and the stiffness ease. If the pain worsens and your back becomes stiffer, stop working on it and seek medical help.
- Is the pain one of aching muscles resulting from the previous day's play or work-out? If so, it should disappear within 48 hours and you can be happy that you have strengthened the muscle a little. Next time you do the same amount of exercise, the effect should be less.
- Has the pain suddenly occurred, or is it gradually getting worse every day, occurring regularly during normal movement? Is it disturbing your rest at night? Do you have limb pain, pins and needles or numbness? If so, this is the time when you must have all your antennae out, cease all physical stress, rest if necessary, put back care at the top of your priorities, and seek medical advice.

No specific advice or rule can be handed out without individual examination. Initially you need to be your own examiner and therapist, gently experimenting with positions while you monitor the pain, never repeating anything that increases your pain *after* you have stopped the action. The choice of remedial positions depends entirely on the pattern of your pain.

If the pain persists or if it is severe, especially if there is referred limb pain with paraesthesia and anaesthesia, you should always see a doctor.

After recovery from a period of back pain it is as negative to feel you 'can't do what you used to' in everyday living as it is to return blindly to all previous thoughtless activities and poor postural habits. Having done all you can to restore normal movement, you must then return to normal living, with back care as part of life. However, if painful episodes have been a recurrent feature of your life, then a change of some part of your lifestyle might be sensible; you may need to compromise over risky activities such as contact sports or jobs entailing heavy manual work; restoring function does not mean continuing with risk. You must do all you can to avoid repetition without wrapping yourself in cotton wool. Prevention means full *use* without *abuse*.

If you are lucky enough never to have experienced back pain, be thankful, but do not be foolhardy. Take note of all the stress-related factors, especially the 'risk situations' on p. 113, and look after your back as carefully as you do any other part of your body.

List of Useful Addresses

National Back Pain Association, 31 Park Road, Teddington, TW11 0AB. Tel: 081 977 5474

The Chartered Society of Physiotherapy, 14 Bedford Row, London, WC1R 4ED. Tel: 071 242 1841

The Ergonomics Society, Devonshire House, Devonshire Square, Loughborough, Leics., LE11 3DW

Institute for Occupational Ergonomics, University of Nottingham, Nottingham, NG7 2RD

Ergonomic Unit, University College London, Gower Street, London, WC1

Ergonomics Research Unit, Robens Institute, University of Surrey, Guildford, Surrey, DU2 5HX

Ergonomics Information Analysis Centre, The University of Birmingham, Human Performance Laboratory, Royal Free Hospital School of Medicine, Pond Street, Hampstead, London NW3

Department of Sports Science, Liverpool Polytechnic

HMSO, 49 High Holborn, London WC1V 6HB. Tel: 071 873 0011

The Health and Safety Information Centre, Broad Lane, Sheffield, S3 7HQ. Tel: 0742 892345

British Chiropractic Association, Premier House, 10 Greycoat Place, London SW1P 1SB, Tel: 071 222 8866

or
Matthew Bennett, British Chiropractic Association, Equity House, 29 Whitley Street, Reading, RG2 0EG. Tel: 0273 774 114

The General Council and Register of Osteopaths, 56 London Street, Reading, Berkshire, RG1 4SQ. Tel: 0734 576585

Munro and Forster, Public Relations (for the General Council of Osteopaths), 37 Soho Square, London, W1V 5DG. Tel: 071 439 7177

The National Bed Federation Ltd., 251 Brompton Road, London, SW3 2EZ. Tel: 071 589 4888

Special Information:
The Health and Safety Executives "Seating at Work" HS (G) 57. HMSO and booksellers reference ISBN 0 11 885431 3

HSE "Manual Handling. Guidance on Regulations" 1992. ISBN 0 11 886335 5

HSE HSC's Health Services Advisory Committee "Guidance on Manual Handling of Loads in the Health Services" 1992. ISBN 0 11 886345 1

HMSO "Management of Health and Safety at Work Regulations" SI 1992. No 2051 ISBN 0 11 025051 6

Official Journal of the European Communities, 21.6.90, Vol 33 No L156 9-13

Index

S

T

U

V

W

X

Y

Z